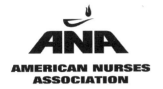

AMERICAN NURSES ASSOCIATION

MW00844776

Implementation Guide to the Safe Patient Handling and Mobility Interprofessional National Standards

Susan Gallagher, PhD, RN

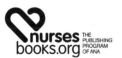

nurses
books.org THE PUBLISHING PROGRAM OF ANA

American Nurses Association
Silver Spring, Maryland
2013

The American Nurses Association (ANA) is a national professional association. This ANA publication—
Implementation Guide to the Safe Patient Handling and Mobility Interprofessional National Standards—
reflects the thinking of the nursing profession on various issues and should be reviewed in conjunction
with state board of nursing policies and practices. State law, rules, and regulations govern the practice of
nursing, while *Implementation Guide to the Safe Patient Handling and Mobility Interprofessional National
Standards* guides nurses in the application of their professional skills and responsibilities.

The SPHM Standards are open, voluntary standards. The standards do not require use of any specific
products or services. ANA does not promote, endorse, or recommend any products or services.

American Nurses Association
8515 Georgia Avenue, Suite 400
Silver Spring, MD 20910-3492
1-800-274-4ANA
www.NursingWorld.org

Published by Nursesbooks.org
The Publishing Program of ANA
www.Nursesbooks.org/

ISBN: 978-1-55810-530-0   SAN: 851-3481   09/2013

First printing: September 2013

Contents

Acknowledgments

I would like to acknowledge Dr. Suzy Harrington for her leadership, support, and vision. I thank Michael, Shannon, and Teresa for your continuing encouragement; Amber, Darla, Eric, Holly, Jaime, and Merl for your valuable contributions and thoughtful insights. I appreciate each of you for the gifts you bring to me and my life. *Thank you!*

—Susan Gallagher

Introduction.

Safety and Quality across Practice Settings: The Emerging Role of Safe Patient Handling and Mobility

In the United States, healthcare workers practice in a culture of sacrifice irrespective of discipline, setting, or specialty. For two centuries blame has been placed on, and typically accepted by, the healthcare worker when injury occurs, despite dangerous working conditions. Just recently, science has helped healthcare workers and other stakeholders recognize the consequences of these unsafe practices. Poor design, unsafe technology, and outdated education and training have all contributed to hazardous conditions and injury. Manual handling and movement have been at the heart of the dangers inherent in the daily activity of healthcare workers.

Experts estimate that the nursing shortage in the United States will increase to a level of 30% shortage by the year 2020. Therapy shortages are documented as well. According to the Bureau of Labor Statistics (BLS, 2012), the demand for physical therapists is expected to grow 27% between 2006 and 2016, and the need for occupational therapists will grow 30% in 2013. The American Physical Therapy Association recently conducted a study citing BLS data (2011) showing that between 13% and 18% of physical therapy jobs were open. Some suggest that the shortages among healthcare occupations are linked to occupational hazards. Research into the impact of musculoskeletal disorders (MSD) on nurses has revealed that 52% of nurses surveyed complain of chronic back pain, while 12% state that they have left nursing because of back pain. A survey conducted by the American Nurses Association (ANA) revealed that one of nurses' top concerns was injury on the job (work-related injury). Many healthcare workers, including nurses and therapists, have high rates of back and shoulder injuries. BLS data reported in 2012 are unchanged from data reported in 2009, which suggest that more than 23,000 lost-time cases of work-related pain are reported each year in the Healthcare and Social Assistance (HCSA) sector; of these, more than 44% were among healthcare support occupations such as aides and assistants (BLS, 2011, 2008).

Nursing aides, orderlies, registered nurses, and licensed practical nurses suffered the highest prevalence (16.6%) of and reported the most annual cases (n = 3,620) of work-related back pain involving days away from work in the

HCSA sector. Unfortunately, the culture has accepted this as the new norm. For example, consider the following quotes from the website of Work Injured Nurses Group USA (WING USA, 2013): "If you're in nursing 10 or 15 years, you'll be hurt. It's a hazard of the trade"; "When the CNA wanted the two of us to pull the 300-pound patient up in bed, I said I'm not doing it. I care about my back and I thought we needed more help. But she said 'I'll do it myself,' and she did." These are simply two examples that illustrate the ongoing acceptance of dangers inherent in the current culture of sacrifice.

Overexertion incidents are the leading source of worker's compensation claims and costs in healthcare settings, with MSDs as the primary outcome associated with such incidents. The single greatest risk factor for MSDs in healthcare workers is manual handling of healthcare recipients. Also contributing to the negative outcomes associated with manual handling is the shortage of nurses. Peter Buerhaus (Buerhaus, Auerbach, & Staiger, 2009), a researcher at Vanderbilt University Medical Center, confirms that in the United States by the year 2025, there will be a shortage of 250,000 nurses. During his career, the late Dr. William Charney (2005, 2011, 2012) argued that without intervention, this problem has endless circularity in that the shortage of healthcare workers leads to increased risk of injury, as described earlier. Workers who experience discomfort, fatigue, overexertion, or pain may work in pain, work while medicated, or simply fail to present to work, thus completing the circle of working shorthanded (absenteeism or presenteeism) and placing other healthcare workers at risk for injury.

Fortunately, solutions do exist. A number of facilities across the United States have begun to integrate the principles of *safe patient handling and mobility* (SPHM) into their safety initiatives. However, a common and widespread misconception is that SPHM technology by itself is sufficient to protect the healthcare worker. Although technology is an important component, technology alone does not support the essence of safety for the healthcare worker and healthcare recipient.

SPHM and Healthcare Workers: An Historical Perspective

In 2000, Audrey Nelson and the teams at the Department of Veterans Affair (VA) Hospital in Tampa, the Tampa Patient Safety Center of Inquiry, and the University of South Florida introduced the First Annual Safe Patient Handling and Movement Conference in Clearwater, Florida. A handful of healthcare workers from a variety of backgrounds attended. Therapists, nurses, dieticians, ergonomists, human factors researchers, insurance stakeholders, and others came together. The value of this interdisciplinary approach was the ability of healthcare workers to discuss, share, and learn from a variety of disciplines. For the first time, many healthcare workers began to understand the limits of body mechanics as a strategy to prevent injury. Further, a number of healthcare workers who previously viewed ergonomics simply as a department within an organization were introduced to the true meaning of ergonomics, and a culture of safety as an essential part of their workday. At that time, few healthcare workers understood that ergonomics is not a new specialty. For example, a good deal of evidence suggests that Greek civilization in the 5th century BCE used ergonomic principles in the design of tools, jobs, and the workplace. In the healthcare setting, an example of this can be found in the description Hippocrates gave of how a surgeon's workplace should be designed and how surgical tools should be arranged. Later, in *Notes on Nursing*, Nightingale (1860) recognized injury as a risk to the nurse while performing an altruistic but dangerous manual handling task.

In those first days of recognizing the challenges inherent in lifting, turning, and repositioning patients, conference attendees learned the special needs of certain patient populations, such as the larger, heavier healthcare recipient. Certain clinical areas, such as the emergency department, surgical services, radiology, maternal health, and others, were identified as high-risk settings and further subsequent discussion provided better understanding of the risks. Additionally, focus on unique clinical tasks, such as hygiene, catheterization, lateral transfers, and others, offered opportunities for conference participants to better address the hazards of caring for the healthcare recipient. To that extent, the emerging Safe Patient Handling and Movement Conference, and increasing awareness of the challenges in creating an evidence-based culture of safety that is designed to improve patient safety outcomes and reduce the frequency and severity of injury among healthcare workers, lent momentum to the overall SPHM efforts.

On June 17, 2005, the State of Texas passed into law TX Senate Bill 1525, the first state legislation requiring hospitals and nursing homes to implement a safe patient handling and movement program. The Texas Nurses Association was instrumental in getting this important legislation passed; it took on effect January 1, 2006. With Texas as the first state to successfully pass such legislation, a number of other states began working toward legislative protection of healthcare workers against preventable injury from manual patient lifting. Since then, nine additional states have passed some level of legislation or resolution, although the laws are inconsistent in content. These states are Ohio, New

York, Washington, Rhode Island, Minnesota, Maryland, New Jersey, Hawaii, and California. H.R. 2480, the "Nurse and Health Care Worker Protection Act of 2013," was introduced to Congress in June 2013. Its aim is to "[d]irect the Secretary of Labor to issue an occupational safety and health standard to reduce injuries to patients, nurses, and all other health care workers by establishing a safe patient handling, mobility, and injury prevention standard," and the text of the proposed bill aligns with *Safe Patient Handling and Mobility: Interprofessional National Standards* (ANA, 2013b).

Although state legislation has focused on the acute, general, and long-term care settings, the healthcare worker of the future will likely work in a number of other settings. For example, today only 20% of physical therapists work in acute care hospitals, whereas 72% of physical therapy assistants and 27% of occupational therapists are employed in acute care. Nearly 30% of nursing jobs are found in acute, general, and long-term care hospitals. However, because of administrative cost cutting, increased workload, and rapid growth of post-acute services, much of the healthcare worker/healthcare recipient experience will occur outside the settings and criteria set forth by many states' legislation or resolutions. Legislative mandates are a great first step, but stakeholders are recognizing the impact of failure to provide adequate methods for safe patient handling and mobility that do not differentiate between practice setting and healthcare workers, and this includes workers in clinics, post-acute care settings, and the home care environment.

Since the first SPHM Conference in 2000, much has happened in the world of healthcare recipient and worker safety. The "Handle with Care" campaign was an ANA initiative. In 2010, the SPHM National Conference was introduced on the West Coast as well as in Florida, thus offering twice-yearly opportunities for interested individuals. Shortly thereafter, a number of national professional associations and publications were introduced. Numerous hospitals, healthcare systems, individuals, and professional organizations offered either regional meetings or pre- or post-conferences at national conferences addressing SPHM. Of interest was the emerging intersection of science pertaining to patient safety and caregiver safety, as well as collaboration between organizations. Consider, for example, the 2009 "Safe Patient Handling Training for Schools of Nursing" curriculum developed in partnership with the National Institute for Occupational Safety and Health (NIOSH), the Veterans Health Administration (VHA), and the American Nurses Association. Further, in 2010, the National Association of Bariatric Nurses formed a task force to examine safe handling and movement as it related to patients of size, and published a best-practice document to present its findings. Other groups showed interest in the topic as well, including surgical services, orthopedic groups, and others. Certification in safe patient handling was made available for the first time in 2012.

Acknowledging Patient Safety Outcomes

A number of national and legislative agencies have identified and monitored patient safety outcomes over the past decade. The Agency for Healthcare Research and Quality, National Database of Nursing Quality Indicators®, and the Centers for Medicare and Medicaid Services (CMS) are discussed herein. However, this list is not exclusive to national and international safety initiatives. The goal of presenting such initiatives is to provide a framework within which to further discuss safe patient handling and mobility as this affects general healthcare safety initiatives.

The Agency for Healthcare Research and Quality (AHRQ) describes Patient Safety Indicators (PSIs) as a set of indicators that provide information on potential complications and adverse events following surgeries, procedures, and childbirth (AHRQ, 2013). The PSIs were developed after a comprehensive literature review, analysis of ICD-9-CM codes, review by a clinician panel, implementation of risk adjustment, and empirical analyses. The PSIs can be used to help facilities identify potential adverse events that might require further study; provide the opportunity to assess the incidence of adverse events and complications using administrative data found in the typical discharge record; and include indicators for complications occurring in a hospital that may represent patient safety events. Indicators also have area-level analogs designed to detect patient safety events on a regional level.

The National Database of Nursing Quality Indicators® (NDNQI®) was established in 1998 as part of ANA's Safety and Quality Initiative, and is currently a program of ANA's National Center for Nursing Quality (ANA, n.d.). The mission of NDNQI is to aid interested parties in patient safety and quality improvement efforts by providing national comparative data to participating hospitals, and conducting research on the relationship of nursing care and patient outcomes. NDNQI is the only national nursing quality measurement program that provides hospitals with unit-level performance comparison reports for state, national, and regional percentile distributions. All indicator data are reported at the nursing-unit level. NDNQI's nursing-sensitive indicators reflect the structure, process, and outcomes of nursing care. For example, critical care units have more hospital-acquired pressure ulcers, rehab units have more patient falls, and nurses working in ambulatory care units have the highest degree of satisfaction.

As part of the Deficit Reduction Act of 2005, CMS recognized what are referred to as hospital-acquired conditions, and placed provisions in the Inpatient Prospective Payment System (IPPS) to allow nonpayment if certain circumstances exist (CMS, 2013b). Health planners are scrambling to find solutions to the nonreimbursable events as described by CMS. Eleven categories of hospital-acquired conditions were included in the IPPS Fiscal Year 2013 Final Rule. Further, the Affordable Care Act added section 1886(q) to the Social Security Act, establishing the Hospital Readmissions Reduction Program, which requires CMS to reduce payments to IPPS hospitals with excessive readmissions, effective for discharges beginning on October 1, 2012. Of the 11 events at risk for nonpayment, at least half were immobility-associated consequences of care. Therefore, the underlying contributing factor in at least half of these events is immobility. So, if members of the healthcare community can manage immobility, we may be able to mitigate some of the economic consequences of these events.

The first immobility-related consequence of care, which is perhaps the most discussed, is the pressure ulcer problem. Pressure ulcers are costly economically, from both a reimbursement and a liability claim perspective. Other immobility-related patient safety issues include: embolic conditions such as deep vein thrombosis (DVT) and pulmonary embolus (PE), hospital-acquired pneumonia, arguably catheter-associated urinary tract infection, arguably surgical site infection, readmission within 30 days, and fall-related injuries. Further, a Joint Commission publication (2012) reported that the issue of falls is a particularly important outcome in healthcare today. In an analysis of more than 7,000 inpatient falls, researchers found that more than 25% resulted in some degree of injury. A number of authors indicate that the safest approach is a safety-based program comprised of trained healthcare workers who use modern mechanical lifts and repositioning devices rather than manual handling. One study documented a 49% reduction in patient falls related to lift and transfer activities using the process just described. These practices also free healthcare workers from the burden of lifting patients so they can devote their energies and mindfulness to direct patient care. The goal is to let the healthcare workers do the health care, and let proper, safe mechanical devices do the lifting. This really is a critical step to protect both healthcare recipients and healthcare workers from injury.

About This Guide:
Some Ways to Implement the SPHM Standards

In 2012, the ANA recognized that despite all the work being done, healthcare recipients and healthcare workers are still getting injured. They recognized the need for consistent, universal, interprofessional, evidence-based standards of care that would be applicable across the continuum of care, and thus convened a group of national subject-matter experts to develop interprofessional national standards. *Safe Patient Handling and Mobility: Interprofessional National Standards* is the result of that endeavor. These eight overarching Standards are organized into two parts: one addresses the responsibilities of the employer or healthcare organization, the other those of healthcare workers. (A substantive part the SPHM Standards publication is its Appendix A, which offers employers numerous strategies and resources for implementing each Standard.)

Implementation Guide to the Safe Patient Handling and Mobility Interprofessional National Standards is a logical next step that complements the standards. The *Implementation Guide* is written for interested individuals who currently do not have a SPHM program or who are in the early stages of developing a program. The *Implementation Guide* offers those individuals the opportunity to get on a fast track to success. Keep in mind that every day without a culture of safety is a day a healthcare worker may experience a career-ending injury. The *Implementation Guide* is designed to work in conjunction with the ANA SPHM Standards publication. Also, the sections following each standard, titled "Evidence: Some Resources and Reading," are designed to provide additional texts to support the "how-to" information included herein.

The *Implementation Guide* is just that: a guide. Interested individuals will still need to begin the journey in a manner uniquely appropriate to themselves, their co-workers, and their organizations. What is universal, however, is the fact that (1) getting started is the most difficult part of the journey; (2) the SPHM program is not the responsibility of an individual; (3) nursing is not exclusively responsible for development or success of the SPHM program.

Within today's healthcare organizations, most employees are working at their maximum capacity, so participating in building a SPHM program compromises their primary function. Most measures in health care are driven by economics—which is understandable to some extent, as organizations cannot maintain viability without fiscal health. To that end, getting started without a strong business case can be a challenge. Even with a team in place, understanding the business case for a SPHM program is confusing; however, without a sound business case for SPHM, program support will arguably be marginal at best. For example, John Celano and others have used statistical models to understand the magnitude of the problem associated with the inability to safely mobilize healthcare recipients. Further, Celano has developed a model to predict future loss based on available data. Most individuals starting programs are not familiar with this type of analysis, but chapter 3 (Celano, 2010) in the comprehensive document *Patient Handling and Movement Assessments: A White Paper*, more commonly referred to as *PHAMA* (Cohen et al., 2010), includes a concise description of the data analysis Celano uses to build a business case for SPHM. The value of the *PHAMA* document is that chapter 3 can be reviewed and used irrespective of the rest of the document.

Data collection and analysis should not become a barrier in developing a SPHM program. For example, organizations already have employees in place to collect and analyze data. Celano and the team at Stanford University Hospitals and Clinics have done this. Risk management, quality improvement, occupational health, and other departments have the information needed to quantify the need for a SPHM program. These stakeholders must be part of the SPHM team, and likely will want to participate in the effort, as this safety initiative serves as a positive measure for their respective initiatives. For example, SPHM initiatives must be aligned with the safety initiatives across the organization because the safety initiatives are tied to economic drivers. Data will certainly be forthcoming if stakeholders understand the benefits of the SPHM program. Consider providing representatives from risk management, quality improvement, and occupational health departments with a link to or a copy of the Celano models in Chapter 3 of the *PHAMA*. A business case is not difficult to build if the right supporters are in place. Further, over time, stakeholders, as part of the team, can present summaries of ongoing data and the SPHM team can formulate a plan based on the data.

If data identification is a challenge, consider the following option. Develop a single-page, at-a-glance tool, titled "Who can get me what I want?," comprised of five columns: Department, Title, Name, Expectation, and Contact Information. Identify the information that is needed; this is the expectation.

For example, consider pressure ulcer development. The expectation is to locate data on measurable pressure ulcer frequency and severity. The SPHM team will assume that the department is nursing or therapy; the title of the person may be wound care clinician, for example; and the name and contact are as yet unknown. In one case, it was not the wound care clinician who managed the data, it was a therapist who had a particular talent for data collection and management. In this exemplar case, although the wound care clinician was a key stakeholder on the SPHM team, for purposes of data reporting it was the therapists who had the information who were named in the tool, "Who can get me what I want?" One SPHM representative in the early phases used the *PHAMA* to identify indicators and then took the tool with him everywhere he went, taking opportunities to ask those around him who was the best resource to locate necessary data. Keep in mind that, arguably, all data exist and will become available as soon as keepers of the data understand how a SPHM program will help stakeholders meet their quality, safety, and cost goals. Never let the fear of data collection interfere with getting started on the journey to a meaningful SPHM program.

The *Implementation Guide* is to be used as a reference guide for implementing the SPHM Standards, not as a book to be read chapter by chapter in numerical order. To that end, each chapter is structured identically to make it easier to dip in and out as you and others at your facility develop or refine your SPHM program. Components include the following:

- An introductory section is provided to frame the context in which to explore the specific SPHM Standard. Case studies, lived experiences, and the latest information and data from literature and research are included.

- Ideas and insights for implementing the standards are addressed from both the employer and the healthcare worker perspectives. Although this guide calls for a partnership between these two primary stakeholders, the rights and responsibilities of each are set forth to better manage expectations with the unified goal of SPHM in mind.

- Resources and readings that provide an evidential basis for the implementation ideas and insights follow each section. Look to the latest research, practical ideas, and an historical context to build a deeper understanding of SPHM across units, disciplines, facilities, and time.

- A case-study approach is included to highlight SPHM issues specific to a community setting. The goal of this feature is to address issues and opportunities inherent in a SPHM program that transcends practice settings.

Each facility will customize *Safe Patient Handling and Mobility: Interprofessional National Standards* to best suit the unique needs of its organization, practice setting, or discipline. The goal of the *Implementation Guide* is to provide a set of step-by-step tools for individuals or teams to begin the journey toward a robust SPHM program. To that end, it includes discussion of barriers to change, tips for championing the project, and ways to best start a SPHM dialogue with both healthcare recipients and healthcare workers.

Evidence: Resources and Reading

Agency for Healthcare Research and Quality (AHRQ). *Patient safety indicators.* Retrieved June 21, 2013, from http://qualityindicators.ahrq.gov/Modules/psi_ resources.aspx

American Nurses Association. (n.d.). *NDNQI home page.* Retrieved August 26, 2013, from http://www.nursingquality.org/

American Nurses Association. (2013). *Safe patient handling and mobility: Interprofessional national standards.* Silver Spring, MD: Nursesbooks.org.

Buerhaus, P. I., Auerbach, D. I., & Staiger, D. O. (2009). The recent surge in nurse employment: Causes and implications. *Health Affairs, 28*(4), 657-668.

Bureau of Labor Statistics, U.S. Department of Labor. (2008). *Number of nonfatal occupational injuries and illnesses involving days away from work by industry and selected natures of injury or illness, private industry.* Retrieved May 22, 2013, from http://www.bls.gov/iif/oshwc/osh/case/ostb2455.pdf

Bureau of Labor Statistics, U.S. Department of Labor. (2009). *Number of nonfatal occupational injuries and illnesses involving days away from work by industry and selected natures of injury or illness, private industry.* Retrieved May 22, 2013, from http://www.bls.gov/iif/oshwc/osh/case/ostb2455.pdf

Bureau of Labor Statistics, U.S. Department of Labor. (2011). *Nonfatal occupational injuries and illnesses requiring days away from work.* Retrieved July 22, 2013, from http://www.bls.gov/news.release/osh2.nr0.htm

Bureau of Labor Statistics, U.S. Department of Labor. (2012). *Occupational health outlook: Physical therapist assistants and aides.* Retrieved August 26, 2013, from http://www.bls.gov/ooh/Healthcare/Physical-therapist-assistants-and-aides.htm

Celano, J. N. (2010). Establishing the business case—Understanding and increasing the value of a PHAMP at your institution. In Cohen et al. (Eds.), *Patient handling and movement assessments: A white paper.* Dallas, TX: Facility Guidelines Institute.

Centers for Medicare and Medicaid Services (CMS). (2013a). *Readmissions reduction program.* Retrieved July 21, 2013, from http://www.cms.gov/Medicare/ Medicare-Fee-for-Service-Payment/AcuteInpatientPPS/Readmissions-Reduction-Program.html

Centers for Medicare and Medicaid Services (CMS). (2013b). *Hospital-acquired conditions (HAC) in acute inpatient payment system (IPPS) hospitals.* Retrieved August 26 from http://www.cms.gov/Medicare/Medicare-Fee-for-Service-Payment/HospitalAcqCond/downloads/hacfactsheet.pdf

Charney, W. (2005). The need to legislate the health-care industry in the state of Washington to protect health-care workers from back injury. *Journal of Long-Term Effects of Medical Implant, 15*(5), 567-572.

Charney, W. (2011). *Handbook of modern hospital safety.* Boca Raton, FL: CRC Press.

Charney, W. (2012). *Epidemic of medical errors and hospital-acquired infections.* Boca Raton, Fl: CRC Press.

Charney, W., & Schirmer, J. (2007). Nursing injury rates and negative patient outcomes: Connecting the dots. *AAOHN Journal, 5*(11), 1-6, 17.

Cohen, M. A., Green, D. A., Nelson, G. G., Leib, R., Matz, M. A., et al. (2010). *Patient handling and movement assessments: A white paper* (Prepared by the 2010 Health Guidelines Revision Committee Specialty Subcommittee on Patient Movement). Dallas, TX: Facility Guidelines Institute. Retrieved August 7, 2013, from http://www.fgiguidelines.org/pdfs/FGI_PHAMA_whitepaper_042810.pdf

Donabedian, A. (1988). The quality of care. *Journal of the American Medical Association 260*(12), 1743-1748.

Edlich, R. F., Hudson M. A., Buschbacher, R. M., Winters, K. L., Britt, L. D., Cox, M. J., ... & Falwell, R. J. (2005). Devastating injuries in healthcare workers: Description of the crisis and legislative solution to the epidemic of back injury from patient lifting. *Journal of Long-Term Effects of Medical Implant, 15*(2), 225-241.

Flegal, K. M., Carroll, M. D., Ogden, C. L., & Curtin, L. R. (2010). Prevalence and trends in obesity among U.S. adults, 1999-2008. *Journal of the American Medical Association, 303*(3), 235-241.

Gallagher, S. M. (2011). Exploring the relationship between obesity, patient safety, and caregiver injury. *American Journal of SPHM, 1*(2), 8-12.

Gallagher, S. M. (2012). Safety, the nursing shortage and the bariatric nurse: Is this an ethical debate? *Bariatric Nursing & Surgical Patient Care, 7*(1), 10-12.

Hudson, M. A. (2005). Texas passes first law for safe patient handling in America: Landmark legislation protects health-care workers and patients from injury related to manual patient lifting. *Journal of Long-Term Effects of Medical Implants, 15*(5), 559-566.

The Joint Commission (TJC). (2012). 2011–2012 *national patient safety goals.* Retrieved from http://www.jointcommission.org/assets/1/18/2011-2012_npsg_presentation_final_8-4-11.pdf

Nightingale, F. (1860). *Notes on nursing.* New York: D. Appleton & Co. Retrieved June 20, 2013, from http://books.google.com/books?id=fAAIAAAAIAAJ&pg=PA3&dq=notes+on+nursing

Reducing nursing injuries. Retrieved June 1, 2013, from http://individual.utoronto.ca/anamjitsivia/nursesrfp.pdf

Work Injured Nurses Group USA (WING USA). (2013). Retrieved August 7, 2013, from http://www.wingusa.org/

Standard 1. SPHM and a Culture of Safety

Many of my co-workers are beginning to feel that we do not need to expose ourselves to the hazards of lifting any more than we need to expose ourselves to blood and body fluids.

Standard 1. Establish a Culture of Safety

The employer and healthcare workers partner to establish a culture of safety that encompasses the core values and behaviors resulting from a collective and sustained commitment by organizational leadership, managers, healthcare workers, and ancillary/support staff to emphasize safety over competing goals.

Moving an Organization Toward a Culture of Safety

In early 2013, when rounding at a 180-bed long-term care facility, the consultant asked Kari, the care associate, how she would transfer a well-known resident, Mr. S, from wheelchair to bed. Mr. S requires maximum assistance, which means that he is able to do 25% or less of the work required for the transfer. Mr. S needs maximal support in the transfer. He can bear very little weight when standing and generally requires a two-person, mechanically assisted transfer. Kari paused briefly in response to the questions, and then spoke with certainty: "I would use the lift." Upon further exploration, Kari explained that a coach was available to help with residents who met certain mobility (immobility) criteria. Kari said that she had participated in care enough times with the mobility coach and Mr. S that she was perfectly comfortable performing the task safely. This is an example of a culture of safety, in which safety is the overriding factor in making choices about tasks in the healthcare setting.

A culture of safety is at the heart of a safe patient handling and mobility program. The challenge to healthcare workers and other stakeholders is that there is widespread misunderstanding about the structure and process necessary for a meaningful program. Introduction of technology, training, policies, and procedures is a great first step, but does not guarantee a culture of safety. The challenge is to transform a program into a culture of safety.

A number of factors affect the ability for a culture of safety to emerge from the necessary structure. For example, consider Julie Lavezzo and Ryan Rodriguez at Marin General Hospital in northern California. In a recent publication (Lavezzo & Rodriguez, 2013), these authors explain that, despite appropriate SPHM structure and improvement in loss history/injury data, they felt there were opportunities to improve the overall culture of safety. A humanistic component was introduced which transformed the program. A follow-up study further suggested that this addition improved satisfaction of the healthcare recipient, and deepened the integration of the SPHM program into the desired patient-care culture of the organization.

Most research suggests that employers and healthcare workers must partner to establish a culture of safety that encompasses the organization's core values and behaviors. The value of administrative support cannot be overlooked as facilities seek sustained attitude and behavior change over time. For example, consider Carys Price at Christiana Hospital in Wilmington, Delaware. Ms. Price explains that the partnership between stakeholders at Christiana Hospital illustrates the successes that can be achieved by offering real-life, practical SPHM practices that meet the organization's economic needs as well as core values. At Christiana, SPHM is integrated into every service line and recognized as a key initiative facility-wide by discussing, communicating, and presenting the topic of SPHM (Price, 2012).

Further, in an environment of competing interests, the value of SPHM must be recognized from a diverse economic and humanistic perspective. In both of the preceding examples, the SPHM program became a culture because the element of safety was integrated into every discipline and unit. The impact of a safety initiative that influences the goals and objectives of healthcare organizations today is essential. A SPHM program will truly be successful only when the program transforms into a culture of safety.

Implementation Insights and Ideas for Standard 1

What follows are selected ideas and insights on implementing the SPHM standard on establishing a culture of safety. They are organized by the sets and subsets of the standards that are required by any facility: one specific to your organization as an employer, the other to your facility's interprofessional healthcare workers. Here we include ideas for developing a written statement outlining the organization's commitment to a culture of safety, supported by appropriate staffing levels, communication, collaboration, reporting, and a process to identify and refuse to participate in care that threatens the health, safety, or well-being of the healthcare worker or healthcare recipient. (See the sample right to refuse policy and procedure in Appendix A.) The goal of this standard is to set the foundation from which the paradigm shift springs.

1.1 EMPLOYER STANDARDS

1.1.1 Establish a statement of commitment to a culture of safety

Implementing Standard 1.1.1

- Recognize the value of aligning this effort with the quality improvement service of the institution, because this service line is responsible for safety and quality initiatives throughout the organization.
- Provide formal training to healthcare workers and other employees as to the meaning of "culture of safety" in order to understand the presence of a safety culture:
  - Identify the current culture.
  - Identify the reasons for the current culture.
  - Communicate why a culture of safety is important to healthcare workers by sharing early success stories through newsletters, bulletins, and verbal communications.
- Identify economic support for a task force, which is charged with:
  - A written commitment to the culture of safety, which will be the cornerstone for resource allocation, policies, and procedures.
  - Ensuring administrative written approval of the document, once completed.
- Reach out to organizational leaders, stakeholders, and frontline employees to identify 8 to 10 individuals, such as nurses, therapists, assistants, and ancillary staff members from different practice areas within the organization (do not disregard subacute opportunities, which include individuals who have direct or indirect contact with the healthcare recipient) who may be interested in:
  - SPHM.
  - Caregiver safety and prevention of injury.
  - Generally recognized safety culture.
  - Behavioral or organizational culture change.
  - Other relevant interest (see Standard 2.1.1 for a more detailed account of this subheading).

- Organize an interdisciplinary team comprised of the identified, interested individuals from a variety of disciplines, experience, or practice settings.
- Create a task force charter consistent with those of other organization teams.
- Develop a 10-item culture of safety written commitment document, comprised of a checklist identifying those behaviors that support overriding safety.
- Obtain administrative approval for the culture of safety written commitment through established organizational channels, using the organizational charts or other structure for communicating information.

1.1.2 Establish a nonpunitive environment
Implementing Standard 1.1.2

- Integrate the institution's risk management service by involving a representative from the risk management team.
- Establish a facility-wide process for managing hazards in a nonpunitive environment by clearly identifying steps to address hazards and establishing a corresponding action plan.
- Identify a current administrative hierarchy/organizational chart.
  - Alter or flatten the hierarchy as it suits the situation.
- Establish a system to improve interpersonal relationships, such as providing relationship training, collaborating with the customer service.
- Recognize the value of "mindfulness" in healthcare workers, including:
  - Concern about errors even in successful systems.
  - Deference to experts, regardless of rank or status.
  - Commitment to resilience.
  - Sensitivity to operations.
  - Willingness to identify and examine system and individual weaknesses.
  - Eagerness to learn and improve by examining weaknesses.
  - Willingness and ability to seek assistance when concerned about a threat to quality or safety.
- Provide healthcare worker support when workers share concerns.

1.1.3 Provide a system for right of refusal
Implementing Standard 1.1.3

- Integrate/adapt the Right to Refuse sample policy and procedure in addressing nurse and other healthcare worker refusal (see Standard 1.1.4).
- Recognize the value of risk management, quality improvement, members of the organization's legal team, and patient care services.

- Establish an interdisciplinary team as described in Standard 1.1.1.
- Establish a written policy that describes the meaning of "right to refuse."
  - Use clear and concise language in the written policy.
  - Use language that includes all healthcare workers or employees who may be at risk or be placed in an unsafe situation, including, but not limited to, patient care associates, radiology technicians, home health aides, volunteers, and members of the valet parking service team.
- Post the Right to Refuse policy in highly visible locations, such as on the inside of bathroom stall doors, in break room and common areas, and in policy and procedure manuals. The Right to Refuse policy should be given to any healthcare workers caring for a healthcare recipient who poses risk, such as a highly rigid or obese healthcare recipient. This conversation may happen with the charge nurse so as to create an awareness of safety for both the healthcare worker and the healthcare recipient.
- Create a written procedure describing safe and meaningful ways to invoke the right to refuse:
  - Identify situations that are unsafe to healthcare worker, healthcare recipient, or both.
  - Ensure proper reporting methods, both immediate and long term, such as written processes; ensure that reports are directed to appropriate individuals.
  - Outline appropriate follow-up of right to refuse actions, such as an after-action review or an alternate facility-specific investigation process.

1.1.4 Provide safe levels of staffing
Implementing Standard 1.1.4
- Integrate/adapt the ANA 2012 Principles for Safe Staffing into staffing for the healthcare worker, irrespective of practice setting or discipline:
  - Safe levels of staffing should be established with input from frontline healthcare workers.
  - Consider the number of healthcare recipients and level and intensity of care to be provided, with consideration given to admissions, discharges, and transfers that healthcare workers must manage.
  - Staffing should consider architectural or geographic barriers regardless of practice setting; for example, the home care worker who must drive long distances between healthcare recipients, as this poses barriers to the actual numbers of individuals who may be treated in a day.

- Consider the location of available SPHM technology and the time required to access that technology.
- Staffing levels should reflect the level of preparation and experience of the healthcare workers who are or will be providing care.
- Staffing levels should reflect the staffing recommendations of discipline-specific professional organizations.
- Ensure that a healthcare worker is not assigned to work in a particular area before that worker's ability to provide care and establish confidence in such an area has been established.

■ Establish a written policy under which a healthcare worker may refuse an assignment when the patient assignment does not match the healthcare worker's knowledge and competencies.

- Create a practice model that matches healthcare recipient needs with the healthcare workers' competencies. For example, staffing needs must be determined based on an analysis of healthcare consumer status, such as the degree of stability, intensity, and acuity; and the environment in which the care is provided.
- Consider professional characteristics, skill set, and mix of the staff, and previous staffing patterns that have been shown to improve outcomes.
- Train healthcare workers on the policy regarding the right to refuse an assignment at annual safety training or department-specific meetings/ updates.
- Incorporate a routine policy review at annual competency or performance reviews.

■ Establish a retaliation-free environment/process for healthcare workers to question the appropriateness/safety of staffing assignments.

- Establish a process to evaluate individual assignment situations cited by healthcare workers, such as matching the appropriate worker with the appropriate healthcare recipient. The charge nurse or individual responsible for assigning workers needs to be aware of the worker's education level and physical limitations. This does not mean that the 5-foot, 100-pound worker always gets the lighter healthcare recipient or easier assignment and everyone else has to struggle with heavy patients or difficult assignments. The ideal is that all workers have adequate SPHM technology, training, and support to provide a safe environment of care for both the healthcare worker and the healthcare recipient.

■ Establish an action plan for unexpected periods of increased activity and/ or acuity.
  ● Develop a written management protocol outlining management responses to the healthcare worker's invocation of the right to refuse an overtime mandate, which may lead to unsafe practices such as working while stressed or fatigued and thus place the healthcare worker and healthcare recipient at risk for injury.
■ Review and evaluate errors and near misses in relation to staffing variables present at the time of the event. Members of the management and leadership team must understand that time is a barrier to compliance. No matter how the job is framed, recognize that healthcare workers are constantly being tasked with more and more, whether it is policy and procedure knowledge and compliance, knowledge and use of SPHM equipment, a new form of charting, sharps disposal, and so on. All these and more are factors that contribute to errors.
■ Seek out new technologies to improve healthcare worker and healthcare recipient safety.

1.1.5 Establish a system for communication and collaboration
Implementing Standard 1.1.5
■ Identify key stakeholders, by title, in the SPHM effort. Keep in mind that each individual title has set goals and accountability to the individual to whom the person with that title reports. Within a healthcare organization, there are a number of interpersonal relationships, and as the program unfolds it becomes important to link the goals of the individuals and individual departments with the goals of the SPHM program. For example, consider a hospital receiving Magnet® status due to higher patient satisfaction scores or a long-term care facility that has addressed adverse outcomes which are subject to fines and nonreimbursement status.
  ● Organizational stakeholders include members of the management and leadership teams, which may use the following titles: CNO, CFO, COO, CHR, risk management, quality improvement, and others.
  ● Unit-specific stakeholders include members of the management and clinical unit-based teams, which may use the following titles: department manager, charge nurse, home care lead team, and others.
  ● Discipline-specific stakeholders include members of specific professions or groups, which may be called home health aides, registered nurses, therapists, dieticians, EMS workers, and others.

- Establish a culture that encourages questions.
  - Include critical thinking skills when discussing the healthcare recipient.
  - Healthcare workers should scrutinize and question SPHM information by recognizing and practicing communication that is open to debate. For example, consider the mobility status of a healthcare recipient: in most cases the healthcare worker must assess and reassess mobility constantly, as it can change in a matter of minutes. Simply asking the healthcare recipient, a family member, or another healthcare worker may not ensure safe mobility practices. However, establishing a culture that encourages questions enhances the health of the worker, the recipient, and the organization.
  - Healthcare workers should expect to receive all key information about their assignment and the healthcare recipient.
  - Encourage transparency by establishing a strategy for two-way discussion pertaining to any additional questions/ideas by socializing the importance of SPHM and then making decisions based on the data that have been developed in healthy, meaningful two-way discussion.
- Recognize the value of marketing efforts in communicating a SPHM program to various individuals, including:
  - Communication to healthcare recipients, visitors, and family members (see Standard 5.1.6).
  - Communication to facility consultants.
  - Communication to members of the interprofessional team.

1.2 HEALTHCARE WORKER STANDARDS

1.2.1 Participate in creating and maintaining a culture of safety

Implementing Standard 1.2.1

- The healthcare worker has a professional obligation to raise concerns regarding any assignment that puts the healthcare recipient or worker at risk for harm.
  - Recognize experiential limitations when deciding whether the healthcare worker has the experience to carry out an assigned mobility task; for example, establish whether a newly hired home health aide really understands how to assist a morbidly obese individual into the shower at home for the first time after having short-stay surgery.
  - Recognize knowledge limitations that may preclude a healthcare worker from fully understanding the dangers inherent in an unsafe practice.

- Recognize skill limitations, especially if the healthcare worker has not had the opportunity to return-demonstrate use of technology.
- Recognize physical limitations that may reduce the amount of weight the worker may lift, push, or pull.
- Recognize language barriers that interfere with understanding the skills necessary for an assignment.
- Recognize cultural differences that may result in feelings of inadequacy if the worker is required to ask for assistance.
- Inappropriate staffing ratios should be addressed, in part, by referring to the ANA Principles of Safe Staffing, and recognizing the chain of command within the organization.
- Avoid inappropriate staffing mix of various disciplines (RN, CNA, LPN/LVN, CNS).
- Recognize lack of proper technology, as determined by after-action data, injury data, and confidential reports such as lack of a proper lateral transfer device that led to a fall-related injury.
- Recognize dangers inherent in "floating"; when floating is necessary, the healthcare worker should be assigned to areas with comparable healthcare recipient or skill needs.
- Healthcare workers are responsible to advocate for themselves, their co-workers, and healthcare recipients by creating an expectation and discussing SPHM and what the organization or care environment does to ensure that technology is used. Healthcare worker are also held accountable to provide care that is consistent with safe practice for themselves, co-workers, and the healthcare recipient to move the individual as safely as possible.
- Healthcare workers are responsible for recognizing their level of physical, mental, or emotional fatigue. When workers recognize their own emerging fatigue, they are responsible for communicating, taking a brief break, asking for help with unfamiliar or strenuous tasks, and using SPHM equipment.

- Healthcare workers will exercise clinical judgment when accepting over-time (mandatory or voluntary) determined by policies and procedure, taking into account how well the worker has functioned in the past in the presence of overtime conditions. For example, historically, the worker is more likely to ignore stresses or fatigue and go in to work to help out a colleague on shift even if doing so is against his or her best judgment. A safe healthcare environment discourages this type of sacrifice because research suggests that this leads to errors in SPHM and creates other threats to safety.

1.2.2 Notify the employer of hazards, incidents, near misses, and accidents
Implementing Standard 1.2.2

- Seek out a process for reporting hazards, incidents, near misses, or acci-dents, such as any fall, near fall, combative healthcare recipient, or similar opportunity for improvement.
- Identify and report situations as defined by the employer.
- Recognize the nonpunitive nature of the reporting structure, such as a reporting structure that is based around education and re-education, and is designed to ensure that the healthcare worker is willing to communicate mistakes or errors rather than fail to report situations. Acknowledge the value of a near miss.
  - Establish a process to report and analyze a near miss. For example, consider the healthcare recipient who presented well on initial mobility assessment and then deteriorated so that the healthcare worker had to manually handle the patient but did or did not injure himself or herself. That report should include a list of questions to examine what happened with the healthcare recipient, investigate the issue, and provide the opportunity to educate and re-educate not only the healthcare worker involved but also the healthcare recipient, the recipient's family members, and other healthcare workers.

1.2.3 Use the system to communicate and collaborate
Implementing Standard 1.2.3

- Identify best-practice form of written communication and collaboration:
  - Organization-wide.
  - Unit-specific.
  - Discipline-specific.

- Recognize the value of interprofessional communication training:
  - Knowledge transfer (classroom training).
  - Skill acquisition (practical, scenario, case-based, hands-on training).
- Identify the need for a crucial conversation:
  - Stakes are high.
  - Opinions vary.
  - Emotions run deep.
- Identify steps to crucial conversation:
  - Observe the situation.
  - Accentuate the positive.
  - Question of concern (open-ended).
  - State the consequences.
  - Solution question (open-ended).
  - Get the agreement (clarify).

Considerations for Community Settings: Home Care Settings

Historically, legislative focus has addressed nurses in the general acute care setting. However, a culture of safety is even more essential in the post-acute home care or clinic settings, and transcends disciplines. Consider Anna, a 20-year-old, 380-pound woman who lives at home with her working family. Anna presents with a left, lower, posterior leg pressure ulcer, bilateral hip pressure ulcers, and intertrigo under her breasts. Anna complains of increasing shortness of breath. She spends 80% of her time in a recliner chair. The social worker who is visiting Anna explains that it impossible to help Anna to the bathroom from the recliner, and wonders how the family accomplishes this task without assistive technology.

The community setting provides unique challenges for the correction of hazards. For example, in the home health setting, the healthcare worker is a guest in the home, and the healthcare recipient is typically financially responsible for the environment of care. Hazardous conditions, broken or inappropriate technology, or unreasonable requests must be discussed with the healthcare recipient and reported to the employer. The employer is ultimately responsible for the health of employees and can determine if engineering or other controls are available to correct the hazards, or determine that care cannot be safely provided.

Evidence for Standard 1: Some Resources and Readings

American Nurses Association. (2006a). *Assuring patient safety: The employer's role in promoting healthy nursing work hours for registered nurses in all roles and settings.* Silver Spring, MD: Nursesbooks.org.

American Nurses Association. (2006b). *Assuring patient safety: Registered nurses' responsibility in all roles and settings to guard against working when fatigued.* Silver Spring, MD: Nursesbooks.org.

American Nurses Association. (2103). *Safe patient handling and mobility: Interprofessional national standards.* Silver Spring, MD: Nursesbooks.org.

Campbell, D., & Thompson, M. (2004). Patient safety alert: Safety culture approach guides health system's efforts. *Healthcare Benchmarks in Quality Improvement, 11*(9), 1-2.

Cohen, M. A., Green, D. A., Nelson, G. G., Leib, R., Matz, M. A., et al. (2010). *Patient handling and movement assessments: a white paper* (Prepared by the 2010 Health Guidelines Revision Committee Specialty Subcommittee on Patient Movement). Dallas, TX: Facility Guidelines Institute. Retrieved May 23, 2013, from http://www.fgiguidelines.org/pdfs/FGI_PHAMA_whitepaper_042810.pdf

Cooper, M. D. (2000). Toward a model of safety culture. *Safety Science, 36*, 111-136.

Falone, P. (2009). *101 tough conversations to have with employees: A manager's guide to addressing performance, conduct, and discipline challenges.* New York, NY: AMACOM.

Frankel, A. S., Leonard, M. W., & Denham, C. R. (2006, August). Fair and just culture, team behavior, and leadership engagement: The tools to achieve high reliability. *Health Service Resources, 41*(4), 1690-1709.

Gallagher, S. M., Steadman, A., & Gallagher, S. M. (2010). Tackling tough topics: Successful frontline conversations every time! *Bariatric Times, 7*(6), 1, 5-9.

Glendon, A. L., Clarke, S. G., & McKenna, E. F. (2006). *Human safety and risk management.* Boca Raton, FL: CRC Press.

Grenny, J. Crucial conversations: Where are you stuck? That's where a crucial conversation is waiting. Retrieved May 17, 2013, from http://findarticles.com/p/articles/mi_m0MNT/is_12_57/ai_n6108404/

Guldenmund, F. W. (2000). The nature of safety culture: A review of theory and research. *Safety Science, 34*, 215-257.

Lavezzo, J., & Rodriguez, R. (2013). *Transforming a program into a culture: Exploring the role of the lift coach as the missing element to meaningful safe patient handling and mobility.* Rancho Mirage, CA: Southern California Association Health Risk Managers.

Patient safety: Rights of registered nurses when considering a patient assignment (2009). Retrieved from http://nursingworld.org/rnrightsps

Patterson, K., Grenny, J., McMillan, R., & Switzler, A. (2005). *Crucial confrontations: Tools for resolving broken promises, violated expectations, and bad behavior.* New York, NY: McGraw-Hill.

Rodriguez, R., & Lavezzo, J. (2013). *Uplifted: Giving voice to safe patient handling— Building a caregiver narrative.* Wilmington, DE: Association of Safe Patient Handling Professionals.

Price, C. (2012). Personal communication/conversation with author, November 9, 2012.

Scott, S. (2002). *Fierce Conversations: Achieving success at work and in life one conversation at a time.* New York, NY: Berkeley.

Singer, S. J., & Tucker, A. L. *Creating a culture of safety in hospitals.* Retrieved April 28, 2013, from http://iis-db.stanford.edu/evnts/4218/Creating_Safety_Culture-SSingerRIP.pdf

Work Injured Nurses Group USA (WING USA). (2013). Retrieved August 25, 2013, from http://www.wingusa.org/

Zhani, E. E. (2012) *Joint Commission Center for Transforming Healthcare releases tool to tackle miscommunication among caregivers.* Retrieved May 29, 2013, from http://www.jointcommission.org/center_transforming_healthcare_tst_hoc/

Standard 2. Sustainable SPHM Programs

I'm a doctor. I am concerned with the amount of lifting and pushing the employees do around here. Yesterday, I learned that one of our ICU nurses had back surgery and within 36 hours had re-herniated. When she couldn't void, her doc was saying he thought it was her meds. I asked, "From what I know about cauda equina, can you tell me why it isn't cauda equina?" And she was right back in surgery....
Is there any way to change this?

Standard 2. Implement and Sustain a Safe Patient Handling and Mobility (SPHM) Program

The employer and healthcare workers partner to establish a formal, systematized SPHM program for reducing the risk of injury to healthcare recipients and the risk of injuries and MSDs in healthcare workers, while improving the quality of care.

Setting Up a Sustainable SPHM Program

A culture of safety can emerge only in the presence of a solid SPHM program. An effective SPHM program requires a complex interplay among a number of disciplines and departments. The goal of the program is to create a partnership between employers and healthcare workers that implements and supports safety goals. Interestingly, many facilities seek data on worker's compensation reduction as the primary measure of a successful SPHM program. Yet, at Stanford University hospitals and Clinics, John Celano and Ed Hall indicate that analyzing worker's compensation data alone is simply not enough. Meaningful safety goals are designed not only to reduce the frequency, severity, and cost of healthcare worker injuries, but also to promote safe, quality care to healthcare recipients. Goals should be individualized to meet the mission of the organization or clinical area/unit. Some suggested goals include: create a safer environment and improve quality of life (QOL) for patients, improve the quality of care for patients, decrease patient adverse events related to manual patient handling, encourage reporting of incidents/injuries, create a culture of safety, empower healthcare workers to create a safe working environment, and increase the frequency with which healthcare workers are able to move and mobilize healthcare recipients.

One of the first steps to a successful, formalized SPHM program is to assemble a team of interested individuals from a variety of backgrounds within the organization. Members of the team should have the ability to identify, receive, and analyze baseline loss history/injury data. Facility, unit, and discipline assessments also provide a baseline from a different, but important, perspective. In addition, follow-up assessment to monitor and compare baseline data allows ongoing improvement.

A written SPHM program ought to include goals, objectives, and a plan for ongoing evaluation and compliance. Integrating the eight SPHM Standards serves the goals of safety.

Implementation Ideas and Insights for Standard 2

This section addresses the complexity of developing meaningful interprofessional support by way of teams. What follows are selected ideas and insights on establishing a sustainable SPHM program. The ideas are organized by the sets and subsets of the standards that are required by any facility: one specific to your organization as an employer, the other to your facility's interprofessional healthcare workers. Addressing the challenges of competing claims for resources is discussed, along with specific and practical ideas for managing the hazards of high-risk tasks. Specific methods to design and sustain a facility-appropriate SPHM program are presented.

2.1 EMPLOYER STANDARDS

2.1.1 Designate a group or groups of stakeholders to develop, implement, evaluate, remediate, and maintain a SPHM program

Implementing Standard 2.1.1

■ Incorporate experts from the organization's insurance brokers/stakeholders; because insurance carriers often have dedicated money, this can help with the initial funding of a SPHM program. Such stakeholders can be identified by working with occupational health, risk management, and quality improvement services within the organization. More specifically, keep in mind that each facility will have a representative of its worker's compensation provider assigned to manage its case (facility/organization). This single point of contact will be able to provide an organized four-year (three plus one) loss history detailing every injury sustained in the facility, including patient handling injuries. This insurance "case manager" is often responsible for many facilities, so his or her time will be limited. This is all the more motivation for the insurance representative to provide you with a wealth of data as you implement your SPHM program, as this initiative stabilizes the risk due to workplace injuries in their account. Compared to most other classifications of workplace injuries, patient handling injuries present the likelihood of "shock losses," which are large, unpredictable payouts that are often paid out over years, especially if the worker's claim, for example, includes extensive rehabilitation following a costly surgery. Stabilizing or eliminating this risk is extremely beneficial to the insurance company and offers the facility the opportunity to renegotiate a lower premium without cutting into the insurance provider's net profits. Therefore, consider this opportunity when identifying meaningful relationships for successful SPHM program efforts.

■ Reach out to organizational leaders, stakeholders, and frontline employees to identify 8-10 individuals who are interested in the development of a SPHM program. This is the discovery part of the SPHM program. It involves asking, listening, and connecting with individuals in a way that clarifies roles and responsibilities. Also consider using the "Who can get me what I want?" tool when identifying opportunities for these stakeholders to be included (see the Introduction). Consider the following:

● Any individual who expresses interest in SPHM.

● An employee who is involved in caregiver safety and prevention of injury, such as the occupational health coordinator, who understands the human and economic costs of injury.

● An individual already recognized within the organization's safety culture; this individual will already understand the barriers and opportunities inherent in framing SPHM as a safety initiative.

● Behavioral or organizational culture change agents who may assist in understanding the necessary process to accomplish culture change within the respective organization.

- A representative whose primary responsibility is for the fiscal health of the organization, unit, or discipline will serve as a champion once the business case has been established.
- The risk management team is instrumental in providing data and serves as a champion once successes become measurable.
- The quality improvement team is instrumental in providing data and serves as a champion once successes become measurable.
- A representative from engineering is essential to facilitate installation of technology.
- A representative from materials management (Central Supply Service) is important, as that department is called on to assist with locating appropriate, available, and compatible technology.
- A representative from environmental services is essential, as laundry service is necessary in sling management and more.
- Other relevant and interested parties.
- Organize an interdisciplinary team comprised of these identified, interested individuals from a variety of backgrounds.
- Create a Task Force charter consistent with that of other organizational teams.
- Obtain baseline data:
  - Incidence of MSD.
  - Severity of MSD.
  - Costs of MSD.
  - Number of light/modified/restricted duty days due to handling injuries.
  - Number of lost workdays due to handling injuries.
  - Prevalence of musculoskeletal discomfort in healthcare workers.
  - Adverse patient event: fall-related injuries.
  - Adverse patient event: DVT/PE.
  - Adverse patient event: pneumonia.
  - Adverse patient event: HAPU.
  - Frequency with which healthcare workers are able to mobilize patients.
  - Healthcare worker retention.
  - Readmission within 30 days.
- Determine what goals associated with SPHM are important to stakeholders, such as those aligned with current safety initiatives or high-cost, high-risk, or high-frequency outcome goals.

2.1.2 Perform a comprehensive assessment of SPHM

Implementing Standard 2.1.2

- Assess attitudes and support:
  - Administrative support:
    - Identify economic and resource support; establish who/what departments is/are responsible for financing the SPHM program.
    - Recognize personal support; determine who are the points of contact and who is willing to be a part of the SPHM committee or task force.
  - Healthcare worker:
    - Assess workers' understanding of SPHM goals.
    - Identify any role misunderstandings.
    - Determine compliance with the SPHM technology, policies/procedures, training, and culture.
- Assess whether staffing levels support SPHM goals:
  - Ensure that staffing levels are appropriate (ratio of healthcare workers to healthcare recipients).
  - Ensure that staffing mix is appropriate (ratio of appropriate disciplines, such as RN, LPN/LVN, CNS, CNA).
  - Determine if healthcare workers have opportunities to attend SPHM education and training sessions.
- Assess application of appropriate ergonomic principles:
  - Recognize handling and mobility tasks that stress the body beyond healthy limits, such as (but not limited to) lifting 35 pounds or more of a static load, or lifting a load weighing less than 35 pounds which is awkward, unstable, or moving; portable floor lifts with poorly functioning casters or carpeted floors that create drag or resistance when moving wheeled objects.
  - Identify unit- or discipline-specific handling and mobility hazards, such as limb lifting by the wound care expert to treat the underside of the lower leg in the home care setting, moving the healthcare recipient from a wheelchair to a radiology table in the clinic setting, or early progressive mobility in the critical care setting. Each such scenario poses hazards.
  - Determine whether ergonomic principles are applied to match the healthcare recipient to the handling and mobility task.

- Assess training methods:
  - Determine whether relevant unit- and discipline-specific training is available to healthcare recipients, such as educating healthcare recipients on ways they may become involved with their own mobility in the facility, and maintaining mobility once they are discharged. This education should also be received by family members and/or healthcare workers at the next level of care.
  - Identify healthcare workers who have attended training by title, number, or percent of total; this can be monitored electronically or via written reports.
- Assess physical environment:
  - Identify whether floor coverings are low-resistant.
  - Determine safe door widths. These are usually designated by building codes; however, from a practical perspective, sometimes the door widths must be enlarged to accommodate the needs of special patient populations. For example, in the case of a bariatric-designated room, the door to the patient care room must be wide enough to allow larger equipment to pass easily. A width of 60 inches is considered sufficient to accomplish this goal. Options for a 60-inch opening include a sliding door or a pair of unequal-leaf swinging doors (one door 42 inches wide, the other 18 inches).
  - Identify rooms with thresholds as a danger, because the irregular surfaces at the door thresholds can create a number of problems, such as fall/trip hazards for the healthcare recipient or worker, or difficulty moving equipment safely over this obstacle.
  - Identify room layout and size for various SPHM tasks. For example, determine whether two beds fit in the room, along with a gurney and lateral transfer device, by using a measuring tape to establish if the room layout allows this task.
  - Ensure that technology is conveniently located. This includes technology such as crash carts, ECG carts, SPHM technology, and/or any other technology that requires physical effort to be lifted or pushed (wheeled) into place.
  - Determine whether technology enhances patient dignity by interviewing healthcare workers and recipients, and by monitoring satisfaction surveys and liability claims when appropriate. Further, keep in mind that SPHM education enhances dignity by promoting safe, sensitive care.

- Determine whether technology promotes safety for healthcare recipients and workers by reviewing workers' injury data and patient safety indicators such as NDNQI® and others.
- Assess for compatibility of technology with existing technology. For example, determine whether floor lifts easily interface with the bedframes, endoscopy tables, and/or radiology tables.
- If incompatible technology is in use, ensure that technology is sufficiently labeled (within line of sight).
- Ensure that power sources (outlets and batteries) are available to meet technology needs.
- Ensure that technology storage locations are clearly identified and marked.
- Identify appropriate uses of technology, such as properly placed and positioned slings on a lift device, and proper inflation of air support surfaces for lateral transfers; match technology or combinations of technology to meet the mobility task.
- Identify the type of frame and support surface (bed and mattress), and the mechanical advantages provided.
- Ensure that clear directions, either written or a photo narrative, are provided for cleaning/processing before and after use. Include information such as the description of the equipment; what classifies it as clean or dirty; and the process to clean the technology, equipment, or device. Post these documents in common areas, such as EVS and where the SPHM technology is located.

2.1.3 Develop a written SPHM program, with goals, objectives, and a plan for ongoing evaluation, compliance, and quality improvement
Implementing Standard 2.1.3

- Identify, by title, those individuals who have responsibility, authority, and accountability for developing and implementing the SPHM plan.
- Establish a clear reporting hierarchy to monitor compliance.
- Identify specific federal, state, and local laws and regulations, including pending legislation; this information can be found on the ANA website electronically, in the risk and quality departments within the organization, or through the Department of Health, Occupational Safety and Health Administration, or the Joint Commission.

- Find and use applicable standards, guidelines, and competencies identified by healthcare organizations such as the American Nurses Association, the American Nurses Credentialing Center's Magnet Recognition Program, the Joint Commission, and the American Hospital Association.
- Incorporate steps to yield a written SPHM program:
  - First determine the need for a SPHM program based on the business case model.
  - Create an interprofessional team (see Standard 2.1.1).
  - Confirm leadership support:
    - Establish designated points of contact.
    - Present to whom and how.
    - Secure commitment.
    - Raise priority.
  - Establish buy-in at all levels, creating collective support:
    - Recognize that the leadership team may seek return on investment.
    - Recognize that the management team may seek patient outcome benefits.
    - Recognize that frontline healthcare workers may seek information on work flow, efficiency, satisfaction, and quality patient care.
  - Select preliminary program goals.
  - Introduce the structural components of a SPHM program:
    - Technology policies/procedures.
    - Training.
  - Create and follow a reasonable, attainable timeline:
    - Preliminary timeline.
    - Adjust to conditions based on unforeseen variables, such as workloads or competing initiatives.
    - Maintain a process for accountability by first having conversations that confirm expectations among key stakeholders, which in acute care may include radiology, wound care, intensive care, laundry, environmental services, education, information technology, human resources, or marketing; in home care, stakeholders may include nurses, therapists, home health aides, marketing, human resources, board members, or members of the executive team.
    - Create a succession plan.
    - Keep the project moving forward.

- Integrate the eight SPHM Standards:
  - Standard 1—Establish a culture of safety
  - Standard 2—Implement and sustain a safe patient handling and mobility (SPHM) program
  - Standard 3—Incorporate ergonomic design principles to provide a safe environment of care
  - Standard 4—Select, install, and maintain SPHM technology
  - Standard 5—Establish a system for education, training, and maintaining competence
  - Standard 6—Integrate patient-centered SPHM assessment, plan of care, and use of SPHM technology
  - Standard 7—Include SPHM in reasonable accommodation and post-injury return to work
  - Standard 8—Establish a comprehensive evaluation system
- Establish a process for ongoing evaluation, compliance, and quality improvement:
  - Monitor satisfaction of healthcare worker and recipient.
  - Monitor technology use:
    - Consider technology that tracks technology usage:
      - Use of technology on types of healthcare recipient.
      - Use of technology by specific disciplines
      - Use of technology in specific area.
      - Use of technology during certain times of the day/night
  - Monitor loss history/injury data pertaining to healthcare worker.
  - Monitor healthcare recipient safety data.
- Determine what goals associated with SPHM are *most* important to stakeholders.

2.1.4 Customize and integrate the SPHM program across the continuum of care

Implementing Standard 2.1.4

- Identify patient care settings, within the facility, that pose actual or historical risks based on an analysis of OSHA 300 logs reconciled with the worker's compensation data.
- List unique patient care needs based on specific settings, such as radiology, emergency department, or critical care in acute care settings; consider CNA tasks in the long-term care setting, or routine EMS calls, which likely do not have the processes and equipment necessary for safe transfers and transport.

■ Recognize universal, facility-wide safety needs that transcend practice settings.

2.1.5 Provide funding to implement and sustain the program
Implementing Standard 2.1.5
■ Identify individuals within the organization who understand ways in which a SPHM program can reduce not only worker injury costs, but also organizational costs, by way of better understanding safety concerns pertaining to the healthcare recipient, or other costs such as training costs, retention and recruitment, satisfaction scores (healthcare worker and recipient), and other organization-specific direct and indirect costs.
■ Identify competing claims for available funding sources.
■ Consider the decision analysis approach:
  ● Identify alternatives:
    ▪ Minimal-level SPHM program.
    ▪ Comprehensive, sustainable SPHM program.
    ▪ No SPHM program.
  ● Recognize information/data:
    ▪ Quantitative data (see Standard 2.1.2).
    ▪ Qualitative data.
  ● Identify preferences:
    ▪ Economic preference.
    ▪ Risk preference.
  ● Calculate the impact of each alternative/choice/decision by utilizing internal and external consultants who fully understand and can communicate the economic and humanistic effects of each alternative/choice/decision.
  ● Make a decision based on the identified alternatives.
  ● Benchmark.
  ● Evaluate outcome.
  ● Re-assess.
  ● Adjust action plan accordingly.
■ Recognize the effects of variation on the cost/benefit model.

2.1.6 Identify the essential physical functions and high-risk tasks of jobs
Implementing Standard 2.1.6

- Review facility-specific outcome data, which is reflected in workers' injury data and also available from risk management service:
  - Identify high-risk jobs, such as the CNA in the long-term care facility who is asked to provide a bed-to-chair transfer without proper technology, or the endoscopy technician who does not have the skill or technology to move the healthcare recipient safely from the supine to the prone position on a narrow endoscopy exam table set on a post that does not allow use of a portable floor lift and sling.
- Identify high-risk functions (tasks), both facility-wide and unit-discipline specific, such as performing urinary catheterization on an anesthetized 600-pound woman on the OR table, or providing colostomy care for the frail, elderly, contracted man at home.
- Perform a general literature review seeking activities that put healthcare workers at risk for injury.
- Perform a focused literature review seeking discipline-specific activities that put healthcare workers at risk for injury.

2.1.7 Reduce the physical requirements of high-risk tasks
Implementing Standard 2.1.7

- Design the facility and use technology to remove the SPHM hazard. Eliminate unsafe tasks or substitute safer tasks (e.g., reduce the number of unnecessary bed-to-gurney transfers by engineering on-unit treatments/diagnostics).
- Integrate safe work practices into tasks that have been identified as historically "at-risk" tasks as determined by data analyzed using OSHA 300 logs and worker's compensation data:
  - Identify alternatives that manage the hazards of high-risk tasks, such as providing in-room physical therapy as compared to performing therapy in a therapy department, which may require multiple transfers and transportation to the department.
  - Develop written task-specific policy to offer safe alternative procedures for high-risk tasks, such as lateral transfers in radiology from gurney to radiology table.
  - Identify administrative controls aimed at reducing exposure to hazards, such as monitoring unsafe flooring conditions that may lead to slips, trips, and falls during mobility activities.

- Consider staffing requirements to accommodate patient acuity and census, such as recognizing special patient populations (e.g., the healthcare recipient who is obese, confused, or complex).
- Incorporate the principles of the 2012 ANA Principles for Nurse Staffing in nurse and other healthcare care worker staffing (see 1.14).
- Ensure that healthcare workers get and actually take rest breaks.
- Seek staffing alternatives to mandatory overtime.

2.2 HEALTHCARE WORKER STANDARDS

2.2.1 Participate in the SPHM program

Implementing Standard 2.2.1

- Locate organizational or unit-specific SPHM program policies and procedures.
- Complete surveys to identify opportunities for improving the SPHM program, including technology, training, support, or other ways to strengthen the SPHM program.
- Participate in education opportunities, such as bedside training, annual competency training and education, regional or national SPHM conferences, and/or SPHM webinars.
- Participate in skill acquisition for high-risk tasks, such as proper worker hand placement in lateral transfers, or proper head placement for the healthcare recipient who has a suspected unstable cervical injury and requires lateral transfer.
- Ensure that SPHM policy matches practice.

Considerations for Community Settings: School-Aged Children

Oscar is a nine-year-old, obese boy attending public school in the greater Phoenix, Arizona, area. He was diagnosed with cerebral palsy when he was 10 months old. In the past three years, Oscar has developed issues with mobility and subsequently has gained weight, which has further reduced his mobility. His increasing weight and weight maldistribution have created mobility issues during school, negatively affecting his self-confidence and self-esteem. (The prevalence of obesity in ambulatory children with cerebral palsy has risen over the past decade from 7.7% to 16.5%, an increase similar to that seen in the general pediatric population in the United States. This finding may have a major impact on the general health and functional abilities of children such as Oscar as they reach adult life.) Teachers and other adults at the school at times attempt to assist Oscar by manually lifting him. Last week a 27-year-old male teaching assistant was injured. The school district is evaluating whether the public school setting is appropriate for Oscar. Oscar's social worker is mediating the debate. The healthcare recipient is financially responsible for procurement of SPHM technology in most home, community, and school settings. The coordination of care at the transition, regardless of whether from home to school or other setting, must address mobility needs. A healthcare worker, such as a social worker or primary care provider, can assist by identifying sources of and funding strategies for varying types of SPHM technology. The goal of SPHM technology in the home care setting is to promote independence and mobility while protecting those who support the healthcare recipient. SPHM across the transitions of care is of mounting importance as part of a meaningful SPHM program.

Evidence for Standard 2: Some Resources and Readings

American Nurses Association. (2013a). *ANA principles for nurse staffing, second edition.* Retrieved August 1, 2013, from http://www.nursingworld.org/ MainMenuCategories/EthicsStandards/ThePracticeofProfessionalNursing/ NursingStandards/ANAPrinciples/ANAsPrinciplesofNurseStaffing.pdf.aspx

American Nurses Association. (2103b). *Safe patient handling and mobility: Interprofessional national standards.* Silver Spring, MD: Nursesbooks.org.

Bhattacharya, A., & McGlothlin, J. D. (2012). *Occupational ergonomics: Theory and applications.* Boca Raton, FL: CRC Press.

Caruso, C. C. (2010). Occupational health and safety for nurses benefits patients, too. *Rehabilitation Nursing, 35*(5), 176, 222.

Cohen, M. A., Green, D. A., Nelson, G. G., Leib, R., Matz, M. A., et al. (2010). *Patient handling and movement assessments: A white paper.* (Prepared by the 2010 Health Guidelines Revision Committee Specialty Subcommittee on Patient Movement.) Dallas, TX: Facility Guidelines Institute. Retrieved August 7, 2013, from http://www.fgiguidelines.org/pdfs/FGI_PHAMA_whitepaper_042810.pdf

The Commonwealth of Massachusetts Executive Office of Labor and Workforce Development, Department of Labor Standards. *Patient handling sample program.* Retrieved May 22, 2013, from http://www.mass.gov/lwd/docs/dos/ consult/patienthandlingsampleprogram.pdf

Gallagher, S. (2010). The meaning of safety in caring for the larger, heavier patient. In W. Charney (Ed.), H*andbook of modern hospital safety.* Boca Raton, FL: CRC Press.

Gallagher, S. M. (2011). Exploring the relationship between obesity, patient safety, and caregiver injury. *American Journal of SPHM, 1*(2), 8-12.

Gallagher, S. M. (2012). Special patient populations. In W. Charney (Ed.), *Epidemic of medical errors and hospital-acquired infections.* Boca Raton, FL: CRC Press.

Koppelaar, E., Knibbe, J. J., Miedema, H. S., & Burdorf, A. (2009). Determinants of implementation of primary preventive interventions on patient handling in healthcare: A systematic review. *Occupational & Environmental Medicine, 66*(6), 353-360.

Needleman, J., Buerhaus, P. I., Stewart, M., Zelevinsky, K., & Mattke, S. (2006). Nurse staffing in hospitals: Is there a business case for quality? *Health Affairs, 25*(1), 204-211.

Pana-Cryan, R., Caruso, C. C., & Boiano, J. M. (2009). *The business case for managing worker safety and health* (Department of Health and Human Services, Public Health Service, Centers for Disease Control and Prevention, National Institute for Occupational Safety and Health, DHHS (NIOSH) Publication 2009-139). Morgantown, WV: National Institute for Occupational Safety and Health.

Reference Guidelines for Safe Patient Handling (2000). *Occupational Health and Safety Agency for Healthcare in British Columbia.* Retrieved May 21, 2013, from http://www.washingtonsafepatienthandling.org/images/Reference_Guidelines_for_Safe_Patient_Handling.pdf

Rogozinski, B. M., Davids, J. R., Davis, R. B., Christopher, L. M., Anderson, J. P., Jameson, G. G., & Blackhurst, D. W. (2007). Prevalence of obesity in ambulatory children with cerebral palsy. *Journal of Bone Joint Surgery in America, 89*(11), 2421-2426.

Rose, M. A., Baker, G., Drake, D. J., Engelke, M., McAuliffe, M., Pokorny, M., … Watkins, F. (2006). Nursing staffing requirements for care of morbidly obese patients in the acute care setting. *Bariatric Nursing & Surgical Patient Care, 1*(2), 115-122.

Rose, M. A., Pokorny, M., Waters, W., Watkins, F., Drake, D. J., & Kirkpatrick, M. (2010). Nurses' perception of safety concerns when caring for morbidly obese patients. *Bariatric Nursing & Surgical Patient Care, 5*(3), 243-248.

Schoenfisch, A. L., Lipscomb, H. J., Pompeii, L. A., Myers, D. J., & Dement, J. M. (2013). Workplace safety equals patient safety. *Scandinavian Journal of Work, Environment & Health, 39*(1), 27-36.

Spratt, D., Cowles, C. E., Berguer, R., Dennis, V., Waters, T. R., Rodriguez, M., Spry, C., & Groah, L. (2012). Workplace safety equals patient safety. *AORN Journal, 96*(3), 235-244.

Standard 3. Ergonomic Design Principles in SPHM

We have a lift but the problem is that rooms are too small to get it in here.

Standard 3. Incorporate Ergonomic Design Principles to Provide a Safe Environment of Care

The employer and healthcare workers partner to incorporate ergonomic design principles, such as the Prevention through Design (PtD) national initiative led by the National Institute for Occupational Safety and Health (NIOSH). Ergonomic design principles use a systematized and proactive process to prevent or reduce occupationally related illnesses, fatalities, and exposures by including prevention considerations in all designs that affect individuals in the occupational environment.

Design to Optimize Safety and Human Performance

Recent attention in healthcare has focused on the architectural design of new construction or remodeled healthcare facilities. This attention includes technology and its effect on occupational safety. Federal initiatives, such as the To Err is Human work, are aimed at addressing the problems of safety, which include SPHM. To address SPHM in a meaningful way, fundamental changes in healthcare processes, culture, and the physical environment must be aligned. This alignment should be planned so that healthcare workers, and the resources that support healthcare workers, are set up to promote safety of both the healthcare worker and the healthcare recipient. Facility design of the hospital, with its technology, has not historically considered impact on the quality of care and safety of healthcare recipient or worker. This provides a unique opportunity to use current and emerging evidence to change the physical environment in a way that improves outcomes.

Consider Banner Health, a healthcare system that has developed "Safe Patient Handling Design and Construction" standards. The principles of ergonomic design and integration of SPHM technology are clearly defined within the Banner Health standards. These standards have become a reference point, within Banner Health, during consideration of all new construction projects and remodels. The standardization includes statements such as the following: 50% of all medical-surgical inpatient rooms will have a ceiling lift installed with a designated weight capacity. Each project may have specific considerations for the team to address, but the general expectations for safety, risk avoidance, and standardization are clear and easy for the project managers to interpret. The goal of this approach is to design in such a way as to optimize safety and human performance.

Ergonomic design principles, such as the Banner Health Safe Patient Handling Design and Construction standards, can be used as a systematized and proactive process to prevent or reduce occupationally related illnesses, fatalities, and exposures by including prevention considerations in all designs that affect both the healthcare worker and recipient in the occupational setting. Experts such as cognitive psychologists and others recognize that the physical environment has a significant impact on safety and human performance. Understanding the interrelationships between healthcare workers, the tools they use, and the environment in which they work is critical to safety. This includes the design of facilities, process flow, technology selection and implementation, ongoing education and training, accountability, and accessibility issues. Experts explain that organizational/system factors that can potentially create the conditions conducive for errors are called latent conditions. The design of a patient care room that allows flexibility and can be adapted to meet changing acuity and the care needs of the healthcare recipient has been found in some institutions to lead to fewer errors by controlling for latent conditions. To that end, researchers are investigating variable-acuity rooms. For example, researchers suggest that two different levels of acute care (intensive care and step-down care) could effectively be merged into a single patient care room by making the room acuity adaptable to accommodate the changing needs of patients. The benefits of the variable-acuity rooms/units are numerous, but specific to SPHM are that fewer handoffs and transfers are necessary, and there are quantifiable increases in available time for direct care without additional cost.

Safety design principles, which address safety among healthcare recipients and healthcare workers, include the following:

- Automate where/when possible.
- Design to prevent adverse events such as falls, immobility-related consequences of care, and healthcare worker injury.

- Design for scalability, adaptability, and flexibility.
- Improve accessibility of technology by placing it in close proximity to the healthcare recipient.
- Improve visibility of healthcare worker to healthcare recipient.
- Involve healthcare recipients in their own care.
- Minimize fatigue of healthcare workers.
- Minimize transfers/handoffs of healthcare recipients.
- Reduce noise.
- Standardize processes.

These widely recognized principles are the foundation of a safe environment, as they encourage designs that support the anticipation, identification, and prevention of adverse events. These considerations become essential in today's economic climate. For instance, the burden of occupational injury, illness, and death is still significant. In the United States, 3.8 million individuals experience work-related injuries. The annual direct and indirect costs have been estimated to range from $128 billion to $155 billion. Moreover, the social consequences of occupational morbidity and mortality affect families, communities, and personal mental health. Consider the nameless nurse, who graduated with a BSN on her 21st birthday. Like 50% of nursing students, she sustained a shoulder injury in her last year of nursing school. The neck, shoulder, and arm pain was so great that she was started on muscle relaxants, physical therapy, and painkillers shortly after graduating. By the time she turned 35 years of age, she had enrolled in the state of California's drug diversion program for impaired nurses.

Statistics suggest that 10% of nurses have a drug or alcohol dependency. Although nurses' abuse of drugs and alcohol is roughly equivalent to the general population's dependence on prescription-type medication, use by nurses is higher, and addiction to street drugs such as cocaine and marijuana is much lower, than in the general population. According to the ANA, the most frequently abused substance among nurses is alcohol, followed by amphetamines, opiates (such as fentanyl), sedatives, tranquilizers, and inhalants. The Prevention through Design (PtD) initiative from the National Institute for Occupational Health and Safety (NIOSH) is described, in part, as the practice of anticipating and "designing out" potential occupational safety and health hazards and risks associated with new processes, structures, technology, and tools. Like the principles described earlier, PtD is a method of organizing workflows and processes, and recognizing the business and social benefits of doing so. For a PtD initiative to be successful, it is not enough that design professionals (engineers, architects, industrial designers, etc.) consider occupational safety and health. There is a need for those who purchase technology to insist on specifications that prevent and minimize risks to both the healthcare recipient and the healthcare worker. To some extent, the prevention of occupational morbidity, mortality, and injury through design represents a cultural shift in the way all aspects of work are organized. Consider the physical and mental demands of jobs, and the physical and social manner in which healthcare workers interact with the workplace environment. This changing paradigm shifts the responsibility of SPHM away from individual healthcare workers and encourages a systems approach to safety. A system-based approach recognizes the value of prevention-based designs, systems, and processes.

Implementation Ideas and Insights for Standard 3

What follows are selected ideas and insights for integrating design concepts to optimize safety and human performance. Ergonomics, sometimes referred to as human factors or human engineering, is defined simply as an applied science concerned with designing and arranging equipment, the environment, and workers' use so that the worker and the equipment interact most efficiently and safely in the occupational space provided. Therefore, ergonomics is at the heart of a safe environment of care. The following insights and ideas are organized by the sets and subsets of the standards that are required by any facility: one specific to your organization as an employer, the other to your facility's interprofessional healthcare worker. Ergonomic considerations of construction, remodeling, and redesign are critical factors in the long-term success of a SPHM program. Workflow, high-risk factors, acuity-adaptable space, and other opportunities become essential points of debate, which are best addressed through team input.

3.1 EMPLOYER STANDARDS

3.1.1 Plan for a safe environment of care during new construction and/or renovation

Implementing Standard 3.1.1

■ Develop an interdisciplinary "Design of Construction and Remodeling" task force comprised of individuals who understand flow in the patient care areas (see Standard 2.1.1):
  - Clinical team members.
  - Patient safety.
  - Caregiver safety.

- Quality risk.
- Environmental services.

■ Utilize mapping/LEAN or other approaches to more fully understand work flow. The basis of LEAN is preserving value with less work, and this is best accomplished by understanding steps in processes or by creating a "map" that features steps of a particular task. For example, if slings designed for use with the unit-based lifts are kept in the basement, the LEAN process would help explain why the unit-based floor lifts are not frequently used. By moving (storing) the slings near the lifts, workers are able to preserve value (use the lift and slings more appropriately) with less work. This manufacturing process has been successful in healthcare settings where a better of understanding of motion/activity leads to improved outcomes.

■ Incorporate ergonomic design principles:
  - Identify high-risk tasks as determined by actual loss data based on OSHA 300 logs in conjunction with worker's compensation reports, worker interviews, and other risk data (such after-action reviews not resulting in worker's compensation report or near miss data).
  - Identify high-risk areas (determined as described earlier).
  - Identify high-risk healthcare recipients (determined as described earlier).

■ Design new construction or remodel projects to manage high-risk tasks, areas, and healthcare recipients.

■ Solicit feedback when appropriate by encouraging transparency in exploring methods to identify strengths and opportunities.

■ Identify opportunities for variable-acuity or variable-use designs to reduce physical transfer and handoffs.

3.1.2 Include diverse perspectives related to ergonomic design principles
Implementing Standard 3.1.2

■ Develop a survey tool that captures SPHM and general patient care needs, such as a single-page survey tool that includes closed- and open-ended questions.

■ Collect, analyze, and report data to team members and other stakeholders, such as architects, designers, and members of the clinical advisory team.

■ Integrate feedback from survey tools into all activities of new construction, rebuilding, and remodeling. Examples include door width requirements for facility-specific needs; toilet mounting based on demographics of the community (wall-mounted toilets have a limited weight capacity and can lead to fall-related injuries); or floor coverings that preclude safe use of wheeled technology.

3.2 HEALTHCARE WORKER STANDARDS

3.2.1 Provide input into the design

Implementing Standard 3.2.1

- Healthcare workers will participate in activities related to ergonomic design principles:
  - Encourage peers and other stakeholders to provide input:
    - Recognize safety needs of the healthcare worker.
    - Recognize safety needs of the healthcare recipient.

Considerations for Community Settings: Rehabilitation Center

Jill, a CNA at a small suburban rehabilitation center, explains that the lift and transfer device is kept in a climate-controlled storage facility off the north parking lot. This facility was selected for storage because it is the nearest to the patient care area. Nonetheless, in order to use the lift, Jill must first find the key to the storage facility, report to another staff member, walk the short distance across the parking lot, retrieve the lift, and roll the lift across the parking lot, up the ramp, and onto the unit. From a quality improvement (QI) perspective, or LEAN approach, this task could be mapped out to establish the amount of time and the number of junctures that would interfere with Jill accomplishing her task. Consider the definition of ergonomics described earlier. Is the object (the lift) arranged so that the worker (Jill) and the object (the lift) interact most efficiently and safely? This danger is inherent in a number of practice settings, but is particularly problematic in the community setting. Inability to safely and efficiently access mobility technology because of poor facility design or processes places the healthcare worker and healthcare recipient at risk.

Evidence for Standard 3: Some Resources and Readings

American Institute of Architects (AIA). (2006). *Guidelines for design and construction of health care facilities.* Washington, DC: American Academy of Architecture.

American Nurses Association. (2103). *Safe patient handling and mobility: Interprofessional national standards.* Silver Spring, MD: Nursesbooks.org.

Brown, K. K., & Gallant, D. (2006). Impacting patient outcomes through design: Acuity adaptable care/universal room design. *Critical Care Nursing Quarterly, 29*(4), 326-341.

Cohen, M. A., Green, D. A., Nelson, G. G., Leib, R. Matz, M. A., et al. (2010). *Patient handling and movement assessments: A white paper* (Prepared by the 2010 Health Guidelines Revision Committee Specialty Subcommittee on Patient Movement). Dallas, TX: Facility Guidelines Institute. Retrieved August 7, 2013, from http://www.fgiguidelines.org/pdfs/FGI_PHAMA_whitepaper_042810.pdf

Henriksen, K., Isaacson, S., & Sadler, B. L. (2007). The role of the physical environment in crossing the quality chasm. *Joint Commission Journal of Quality& Patient Safety, 33*(11 Suppl.), 68-80.

Institute of Medicine. (1999). *To err is human: Building a safer health system.* Washington, DC: National Academies Press.

Institute of Medicine. (2004). *Keeping patients safe: Transforming the work environment of nurses.* Washington, DC: National Academies Press.

Joseph, A. (2006). *The role of the physical and social environment in promoting health, safety, and effectiveness in the healthcare workplace.* Concord, CA: Center for Health Design. Retrieved from www.healthdesign.org/research/reports/workplace.php

Knutt, E. (2005). Healthcare design: Build for the future. *Health Services Journal, 115*(5940), 35-37.

Reiling, J. (2006). Safe design of healthcare facilities. *Quality & Safety in Health Care, 15*(Suppl. 1), i34-i40.

Reiling, J., Hughes, R. G., & Murphy, M. R. (2008). *The impact of facility design on patient safety.* Retrieved May 25, 2013, from http://www.ncbi.nlm.nih.gov/pubmed/21328735

Schulte, P. A., Rinehart, R., Okun, A., Geraci, C. L., & Heidel, D. S. (2008). National Prevention through Design (PtD) initiative. *Journal of Safety Research, 39*, 115–121.

Standard 4.
SPHM Technology

After I graduate, I'm going to go work where they have all the ceiling lifts and things.

Standard 4. Select, Install, and Maintain SPHM Technology

The employer and healthcare workers partner to incorporate appropriate SPHM technology for the program. Such a program provides the assistive tools within the organization and at point of care that are used to facilitate SPHM, thus minimizing the risk of injury to both the healthcare recipient and the healthcare worker. SPHM technology may include equipment, devices, accessories, software, and multimedia resources.

The Journey Toward Meaningful SPHM Technology

Communication and collaboration are critical to the overall success of a SPHM program, but are especially important when selecting, installing, and maintaining SPHM technology. Healthcare organizations are challenged to develop and use a variety of communication systems and tools to inform and engage the healthcare worker. Collaboration among leaders, managers, healthcare workers, ancillary/support staff, and healthcare recipients is woven throughout the ANA SPHM Standards.

Seeking input related to real or perceived barriers can increase healthcare worker engagement in using SPHM technology. SPHM research suggests that barriers are more likely to be resolved if addressed prior to implementation of SPHM programs. For example, Sharon is a part-time radiology technician who works at night, and believes that it is important to mention that the quality of the technology should be considered. She explains that some of the lifts are loud, intrusive, bulky, and aesthetically unpleasing. She knows this firsthand because of her night work and the transfers involved with stat radiologic procedures. Sharon explains that the facility where she works has a "quiet at night" delirium prevention initiative. The floor-based lift technology that was initially purchased was so loud, the nurses and transporters were discouraged from using it. Sharon restates that quality should be as much of a consideration as price when considering 24-hour use of equipment.

A baseline assessment designed to identify the healthcare workers' perceptions of risk, pain, and discomfort may help leaders and managers better recognize opportunities to collaborate with healthcare workers in SPHM efforts across units, disciplines, and practice settings by appealing to the healthcare worker's personal concerns. Colleen Burgio at St. Joseph's/Chandler Hospital in Savannah, Georgia, explains that an online employee survey has been helpful in better understanding baseline SPHM tasks and use of technology among healthcare workers at her facilities. The survey Burgio uses serves as an introduction to an organizational SPHM technology needs assessment, from the frontline user's perspective (Burgio, 2013).

Other assessment tools may be helpful, such as a Patient Dependency Assessment or Patient Mobility Assessment. These data are often used to plan technology for an individual healthcare recipient. But consider a point prevalence study, which captures the dependency or mobility status of healthcare recipients on a particular unit. For example, in planning for assistive toileting devices, some facilities recognize that it was not the fully independent or fully dependent patients who were candidates for powered toilets. Rather, it was the partially dependent and partially immobile patients who were best served by this technology. In that case, during planning for equipment, this knowledge helped planning teams understand the number of healthcare recipients who on any one day were partially dependent and partially immobile, and thus a better calculation could be made in ordering such technology. For example, if 50% of healthcare recipients on an orthopedic unit met criteria for this technology and the unit was a 30-bed unit, then one could assume that the planning team would plan to purchase or rent 15 powered toilets. A regularly planned point prevalence survey might be performed quarterly to validate the data over time. Equipment selection and par levels can be an exciting and complex task.

Assessment-based criteria for use of technology, communication for use of SPHM technology, equipment storage, tracking, and maintaining equipment are all essential. Communication is a key element in this process. Common barriers to use of technology include inadequate quantities of SPHM technology, or technology that is difficult to use, incompatible, or improperly cleaned or maintained. Access to SPHM technology is another major barrier. Access issues may result when SPHM technology is located in an inconvenient place or difficult to use due to space restraints. Overcoming barriers requires teamwork across the facility or work setting.

Implementation Ideas and Insights for Standard 4

What follows are selected ideas and insights on implementing the SPHM standard on selecting, installing, and maintaining SPHM technology. The ideas and insights are organized by the sets and subsets of the standards that are required by any facility: one specific to your organization as an employer, the other to your facility's interprofessional healthcare workers. Organizational assessment and creative methods to best test and try out new technology, along with an action plan to introduce and maintain new technology, are part of this section.

4.1 EMPLOYER STANDARDS

4.1.1 Perform an organizational SPHM technology needs assessment
Implementing Standard 4.1.1
- Establish an interdisciplinary task force (see Standard 2.1.1).
- Perform a general literature review to identify universal technology need.
- Establish whether technology is available to the region, facility, or practice setting.
- Perform a unit- or discipline-specific literature review to identify focused technology needs.

4.1.2 Develop a plan for the selection of SPHM technology
Implementing Standard 4.1.1
- Establish a log of technology and devices:
  - Facility-wide.
  - Unit-specific.
  - Discipline-specific.
- Determine compatibility and interoperability of specific technology:
  - Recognize varying weight limits.
  - Develop a system to identify capability and interoperability.

4.1.3 Provide opportunities for trial and provide feedback about SPHM technology
Implementing Standard 4.1.3
- Recognize the value of education department, risk management, quality improvement, clinical staff members, end users, value analysis representative, and others.

- Identify organizational policy for technology trial/feedback:
  - Develop a written plan for technology feedback if a process is not in place; this can be done by way of a single-page description of collecting, analyzing, and reporting technology feedback, including titles of workers involved in this evaluation process.
- Recognize steps in technology selection:
  - Identify a current technology vendor by determining whether constraints exist that preclude use of a particular vendor, such as contracts, geographic location, practice setting, delivery options, and so on.
  - Include members of the SPHM task force (see Standard 1.1.1).
  - Include end users of technology in the evaluation process by identifying the workers who most directly use the technology, such as the radiology technician who uses lateral transfer devices for gurney-to-table transfers, or the EMS worker who uses a stair glide to transport a patient from a second-floor apartment.
  - Identify budget constraints:
    - Differentiate between cost, value, and pricing by creating an economic and clinical model to evaluate barriers or opportunities using a particular technology.
    - Include risk management and quality improvement representatives when possible.
  - Coordinate technology fairs:
    - Promote demonstration opportunities to all healthcare workers.
    - Incorporate opportunities for written and verbal feedback, such as survey tools or direct conversations with end users.
  - Select a limited technology trial per facility policy based on end-user preferences, compatibility with existing equipment, and economic concerns.
- Analyze written and verbal feedback.
- Review the analysis of the written and verbal feedback and present feedback to the decision-making team/task force, using existing communication processes to share compatibility, preferences, and economic impact of prospective technology; consider including a presentation by an end user to discuss qualities of the technology being considered.

4.1.4 Develop a SPHM technology procurement plan and introduction schedule

Implementing Standard 4.1.4

- Assemble a task force for:
  - Technology procurement plan.
  - Introduction schedule, which is based on the familiarity workers have with the technology and the complexity of the technology.
- Consider the following representative departments to serve as members of the task force:
  - Education, for coordination of training on new technology.
  - Engineering, to coordinate any evaluation of installation activities.
  - Risk management, to establish the need for technology from a liability and safety perspective.
  - Quality improvement, to establish the need for technology from a quality and safety perspective.
  - Patient care services, to offer feedback as an end user:
    - Nursing.
    - Therapy.
    - Diagnostic services.
  - Environmental, to coordinate processing of slings and other reusable devices.
  - Distribution, to coordinate distribution and par levels pertaining to technology.
- Determine whether a process is in place to introduce new technology:
  - If no process is currently in place, establish a process for SPHM technology procurement and an introduction plan by benchmarking with similar organizations or departments within the organizations that have provided similar procurement and introduction strategies for like initiatives.
  - Ensure that accountability is in place for the process by first communicating expectations with stakeholders, seeking commitment and accountability.
  - Ensure that data are captured (see below).
- Identify steps toward, and a reasonable and attainable timeline for, the SPHM technology procurement based on the complexity of the technology and organization.
- Identify steps toward, and a reasonable and attainable timeline for, the introduction schedule based on input from marketing, education, and other stakeholders.

- Ensure that combined worker injury data are used to provide focus training:
  - High-risk areas (such as custodial care in the home care or long-term care settings).
  - High-risk tasks (such as early, progressive mobility in critical care).
  - High-risk discipline (such as the CNA in a rehabilitation unit, or the OR tech in a metabolic surgery center).

4.1.5 Provide and strategically place SPHM technology for accessibility
Implementing Standard 4.1.5
- Identify unit- or discipline-specific high-risk tasks based on safety data pertaining to the healthcare worker or recipient (see Standards 3.1.1 and 2.1.1).
- Identify technology that matches tasks.
- Place unit- or discipline-specific technology as near as possible to the task.
- Identify storage opportunities:
  - Ensure access to power source/battery.
  - Provide an organized environment that reflects the importance of storing technology in line of sight, clearly labeled, within reach, and at adequate par levels.
  - Ensure a clear path to the technology.

4.1.6 Install fixed SPHM technology according to manufacturer's specifications
Implementing Standard 4.1.6
- Recognize the value of engineering as the primary resource to reinforce mechanical safety of technology, monitor safe installation according to manufacturer's specifications, and recognize any structural concerns.
- Locate manufacturers' specifications for all SPHM technology.
- Ensure that installation of fixed SPHM adheres to manufacturers' specifications:
  - Evaluate at initial installation.
  - Develop a process to monitor safety at regularly scheduled intervals by first engaging engineering services, or another designee, as a significant stakeholder in the SPHM process, with the goal of integrating safety monitoring of SPHM technology using existing processes for such monitoring.
- Develop provisions for unexpected inoperability of technology, such as repair or removal and replacement of such technology.

4.1.7 Establish a system to clean, disinfect, maintain, repair, and upgrade SPHM technology

Implementing Standard 4.1.7

- Recognize the value of engineering and environmental services to support processes to clean, disinfect, repair, or upgrade technology.
- Identify an existing process to clean and disinfect technology based on manufacturers' internal infection control recommendations
- Identify an existing process to maintain and repair technology.
- Identify an existing process to upgrade technology based on evolving clinical needs and manufacturers' recommendations for longevity; this can be done by first engaging members of the clinical team, engineering service, or other designee, who then collectively establish an open-ended communication process for determining necessary upgrades based on evolving clinical or technology requirements.
- In the absence of appropriate policy/procedure, develop a policy/procedure regarding cleaning, disinfecting, maintaining, repairing, and upgrading technology based on manufacturer's recommendations.
- Identify, by title, who is responsible for monitoring, and acting on, upgrade or recall notices for technology (technology or software); this can be done by first engaging engineering services, or another designee, as a significant stakeholder in the SPHM process, with the goal of managing upgrade or recall notices for technology.

4.2 HEALTHCARE WORKER STANDARDS

4.2.1 Participate in the SPHM technology needs assessment

Implementing Standard 4.2.1

- Report, in writing, unmet SPHM technology needs per policy:
  - Report, in a transparent manner, the impact on healthcare workers in cases such as lack of slide sheets for a 100-pound woman with mobility assessment indicating maximum assistance, who requires in-bed repositioning.
  - Report, in a transparent manner, the impact on the healthcare recipient when a near miss occurs because inadequate sling options are provided.
  - Report, in a transparent manner, the impact on family members when a healthcare recipient with a mobility assessment indicating a need for moderate assistance incurs a fall-related injury, due to lack of a sit-to-stand technology, that requires an extended acute care, rehabilitation, and long-term care experience.

- Report, in a transparent manner, the impact on other employees, such as the laundry service employee who fails to understand proper processing of slings and other technology.
- Report, in writing and per policy, incompatible technology or technology with features that are not interoperable as expected.

4.2.2 Participate in SPHM technology selection
Implementing Standard 4.2.2

- Participate in cost analysis discussions:
  - Recognize risk and quality features of technology, such as a walker with attachments for accessories and devices to better provide early progressive mobility in intensive care.
  - Recognize liability benefits of technology, such as full body lateral rotation as an adjunct to repositioning for purposes of promoting skin health and preventing worker injury.
  - Recognize cost/value of technology, such as the balance of rental compared with purchase of technology.
- Attend technology fair activities.
- Provide candid feedback on SPHM technology.

Considerations for Community Settings: Home Care Setting

Sharon has provided home care in her local community for the past 25 years. She is reminded of the time when she would kneel at the client's feet and rest the client's leg on her shoulder in order to examine and treat a posterior lower leg wound. Today, she carries with her a device that elevates the client's leg mechanically. She is able to assess for any related client discomfort, and Sharon explains that she certainly feels better at the end of the day not having to bear the burden of so much weight manually. A subject-matter expert in SPHM technology can provide solutions for specific problems, or develop solutions for an entire organization. The SPHM technology industry continues to develop new technologies, work practices, and systems to meet the needs of users across the continuum of care. Newer technologies solve age-old problems like narrow doorways, small bathrooms, low beds, and steps. Healthcare recipients and their families must be encouraged to provide input regarding the usability, usefulness, and desirability of the SPHM technology options available to them. Consider Sharon, who never imagined such technology would be available, but is now learning and implementing ways to provide ergonomically sound care regardless of the practice setting.

Evidence for Standard 4: Some Resources and Readings

American Nurses Association. (2103). *Safe patient handling and mobility: Interprofessional national standards*. Silver Spring, MD: Nursesbooks.org.

Burgio, C. (2011). Using the intranet to administer a safe patient handling and movement implementation survey to direct caregivers. *American Journal of SPHM, 1*(1), 14-21.

Burgio, C. (2013). Personal communication/conversation with author, August 9, 2013.

Charney, W. (2011). *Handbook of modern hospital safety*. Boca Raton, FL: CRC Press.

Cohen, M. A., Green, D. A., Nelson, G. G., Leib, R., Matz, M. A., et al. (2010). *Patient handling and movement assessments: A white paper* (Prepared by the 2010 Health Guidelines Revision Committee Specialty Subcommittee on Patient Movement). Dallas, TX: Facility Guidelines Institute. Retrieved August 7, 2013, from http://www.fgiguidelines.org/pdfs/FGI_PHAMA_whitepaper_042810.pdf

Gallagher, S. M. (2011). Exploring the relationship between obesity, patient safety, and caregiver injury. *American Journal of SPHM, 1*(2), 8-12.

Good Shepherd Medical Center (2008). *Safe patient handling & movement resources guide*. Retrieved June 15, 2013, from http://www.hcergo.org/Sample%20SPH%20Resource%20Guide%202011.pdf

Lavezzo, J., & Rodriguez, R. (2013). *Transforming a program into a culture: Exploring the role of the lift coach as the missing element to meaningful safe patient handling and mobility*. Rancho Mirage, CA: Southern California Association of Health Risk Managers.

National Institute for Occupational Safety and Health. *NIOSH program portfolio: Musculoskeletal disorders*. Retrieved June 6, 2013, from http://www.cdc.gov/niosh/programs/msd/

National Quality Forum. *Effective communication and care*. Retrieved June 6, 2013, from http://www.qualityforum.org/Topics/Effective_Communication_and_Care_Coordination.aspx

Nelson, A., & Fragala, G. (2004). Equipment for safe patient handling and movement. In W. Charney & A. Hudson (Eds.), *Back injury among healthcare workers*. Washington, DC: CRC Press.

Perez, A., Rendahl, T., Murray, G., & Monaghan, E. (2012). Safe patient handling and movement: Equipment safety. *American Journal of SPHM, 2*(4), s1-s17.

Pexton, C. *Healthcare quality initiatives: The role of leadership.* Retrieved May 22, 2013, from http://www.isixsigma.com/implementation/change-management-implementation/healthcare-quality-initiatives-role-leadership/

Standard 5. SPHM Education, Training, and Competence

I'm a first-year nursing student. We did clinicals at the nursing home. They had a lift but it was always way down the hall on the next unit over. Now, I realize, we did a lot of lifting we shouldn't have done.

Standard 5. Establish a System for Education, Training, and Maintaining Competence

The employer and healthcare workers partner to establish an effective system of education and training to maintain SPHM competence of healthcare workers and ancillary/support staff.

Simulating Real-World Experiences to Build Confidence and Competence

Historically, many have believed that the purchase of SPHM technology was synonymous with a SPHM program. Time has proven that this is not the case. Audrey Nelson and co-authors (2008) outline the following steps to success: administrative support, policies, procedures, technology, and training. Education and training are key elements to success.

Education is described as knowledge transfer and is essential to sustaining success over time. For example, in years past healthcare workers were told that heavy lifting led to issues of wear-and-tear injuries. Consider William, a healthcare worker who has lifted weights in his garage for 12 years. Although he was told that activities such as the dead lift or deep squats were damaging over time if too many repetitions were performed with excess weight, he was excited about body building, and lifted the maximum amount of weight possible for as many repetitions as his body allowed. Initially, William experienced occasional neck and shoulder pain; today, he explains that he now experiences neck, shoulder, knee, and back pain more than 75% of the time. This discomfort interferes with his sleep and ability to enjoy the activities of everyday life. Anecdotally, healthcare workers, like William, knew that damage from wear-and-tear injuries over time was likely because after certain lifting tasks, the healthcare worker felt fatigue, discomfort, or pain. However, even more problematic is that some healthcare workers, like William, would perform what is now recognized as unsafe handling practices for years with little discomfort, until the damage was done—at which point the consequences became lifelong and severe. However, unlike William, James, a physical therapy assistant at a larger urban acute care hospital, explains that injuries can occur irrespective of one's strength or appearance of strength. James, who is tall and muscular, explains that he is always the first person asked to help move a larger or heavier healthcare recipient, because he has the look of a very strong individual. He explains to other healthcare workers that technology is the first line of defense against injury when performing such tasks, and goes on to explain that if he hurt himself at work he would be unable to participate in the activities he enjoys outside of the work setting. James is a safe, healthy ambassador and champion for the SPHM program and serves as an unofficial trainer as well. The issue, historically, is that healthcare workers did not have evidence that fully described the manner in which cumulative and acute injuries develop.

Researchers now have science to help healthcare workers better understand the dangers inherent in manual handling activities. William Marras at Ohio State University explains that 75% of the time that the healthcare worker lifts more than 35 pounds, a microfracture occurs at the vertebral endplate (Marras, 2008). This microfracture is designed to heal completely, but will produce a small amount of scar tissue. Further, Tom Waters (1999) explains that the 35-pound limit is a maximum, especially when the task is performed under less favorable circumstances, such as: lifting with extended arms, lifting when near the floor, lifting when sitting or kneeling, lifting with one's trunk twisted or with the load off to the side of one's body, lifting with one hand, lifting in a restricted space, and lifting during a shift lasting longer than eight hours. The human body is not designed to lift more than 35 pounds repeatedly throughout the day, the year, or a lifetime, as occurs in the life of today's healthcare worker. This science creates the foundation for education.

Training is described as skill acquisition, and differs from education in that it has a performance component. Some consider education as answering the "why" question, whereas training answers the "how" question. Skill acquisition can occur in a classroom, at the bedside, or in a simulation center or learning lab. Proponents of the simulated experience argue that "Michael Jordan didn't become a great free throw shooter by watching a video of someone else shoot free throws." For this reason, the simulated experience is gaining popularity in SPHM efforts. For example, the Swedish Hospital System in Washington State has had a SPHM Learning Lab, with simulated opportunities, in place for at least five years. The lab is designed to allow healthcare workers to practice with technology in a safe environment. The Banner Health System currently has four learning labs throughout the Banner system. The largest (in Mesa, Arizona) is a converted hospital; this simulation center offers endless opportunities for skill acquisition.

The SPHM Simulation Center at the Immersion and Simulation Based Learning Center at Stanford University in Palo Alto, California, is managed in conjunction with Stanford Hospital and Clinics. This simulation center provides monitored classrooms and a "hands-on" experience. Dr. Gaba, Director of the simulation center, explains that simulation training is a technique, not a technology (Gaba, 2007). Simulation training is designed to replace or amplify real experiences. Interest in simulation training for health care emerged from the successful use of simulation training in nonmedical industries. Examples are commercial and private aviation, the military, and other industries that are hazardous and complex. In the SPHM simulation center, learners experience compatibility between technology, car extractions, and discipline-specific sling selection, which are some (but not all) of the skills also taught at the SPHM simulation center at Stanford. The value of this model is that education and training can occur concurrently. Further, an environment dedicated to simulated techniques allows mistakes to be made in a controlled setting, where issues can be mitigated prior to contact with the healthcare recipient and family members.

Regardless of the structure selected for education and training, it best serves the employer and the healthcare worker to partner in establishing an effective and meaningful system of education and training to maintain SPHM competence.

Implementation Ideas and Insights for Standard 5

What follows are selected ideas and insights on implementing the SPHM standard on establishing a process for knowledge transfer and skill acquisition, within the context of ongoing proficiency. A number of models are presented, each with the goal of supporting a meaningful SPHM program and culture through education, training, and continued opportunities for maintaining competence. The ideas and insights are organized by the sets and subsets of the standards that are required by any facility: one specific to your organization as an employer, the other to your facility's interprofessional healthcare workers.

5.1 EMPLOYER STANDARDS

5.1.1 Establish an education and training system
Implementing Standard 5.1.1

- Recognize the value of the education department, as this department has processes and mechanisms in place to coordinate and integrate SPHM information into new and existing training/education efforts.
- Recognize the difference between education (knowledge transfer) and training (skill acquisition), as the formats for these activities are different. Education generally occurs as a workshop, lecture, or self-directed study module; in contrast, training is best accomplished in a simulation laboratory/center, on-unit hands-on demonstration, and/or return demonstration or workshop.
- Facility orientation:
  - Emphasize the organization's commitment to a culture of safety.
  - Integrate SPHM solutions into facility orientation, such as interactive scenario-based training.
  - Provide evidence pertaining to SPHM, such as the science supporting lift limits or the pathophysiology of back injury.
  - Allow hands-on skill acquisition specific to a practice area.
  - Provide training that specifically explains the therapeutic and mechanical features of the technology, such as bed operations as a means to optimize the mechanical advantage of SPHM practices:
    - Limitations.
    - Therapeutic features.

5.1.2 Include healthcare workers from across the continuum of care
Implementing Standard 5.1.2

- Determine unit-specific hazardous tasks:
  - Identified by healthcare worker feedback/input.
  - Identified in scientific literature.
  - Based on injury data.
- Create "just-in-time" (on-unit, point-of-care, and as-needed) unit-based skill development activities to address unit-specific hazards.

5.1.3 Provide time for employees to participate in learning sessions
Implementing Standard 5.1.3
- Assure adequate time off the unit for education.
- Establish a train-the-trainer (mobility coach/champion), on-unit learning opportunity:
  - Integrate point-of-care training by a lift team member, mobility/lift coach, or unit champion.
  - Monitor skill acquisition.
  - Ensure that workers have hands-on opportunities.
  - Provide unit-, discipline-, or facility-specific training.

5.1.4 Provide appropriate SPHM technology for education and training
Implementing Standard 5.1.4
- Determine whether there is consistency between the technology used for training and the technology available in the actual care areas.
- Consider a meaningful simulation center:
  - Integrate only the use of technology actually available in healthcare recipient care areas.
  - Discard *all* inoperable, incompatible, or outdated technology.
- Encourage point-of-care training as a follow-up to learning sessions and learning in the simulation center.

5.1.5 Require and document healthcare worker competence
Implementing Standard 5.1.5
- Identify a system to document competence:
  - Document attendance at session/courses.
  - Provide hands-on training.
  - Encourage return demonstrations.
  - Provide scenario- or case-based training:
    - Encourage healthcare workers to share examples of challenging tasks.
    - Provide training in ways to mitigate the expressed challenges.
  - Provide on-unit or point-of-care coach/train-the-trainer signoff.
  - Ensure annual competence training; consider including the topic in an annual skills fair.
- Develop a system for unit- or discipline-specific ongoing monitoring:
  - Manage accountability.
  - Manage expectations.

5.1.6 Provide time and resources for education of healthcare recipients
Implementing Standard 5.1.6

- Recognize the value of customer relations, public relations, patient care services, healthcare workers, and others to support education and awareness for the healthcare recipient, family members, and visitors.
- Establish a task force to determine best processes for educating healthcare recipients in SPHM philosophy.
- Develop a written policy describing processes for educating the healthcare recipient, family members, and visitors about the SPHM program; this policy should specifically outline methods for workers to use to describe expectations, which include mobility activities and technology based on assessment of each healthcare recipient's specific mobility needs.
- Consider written/electronic tools to reinforce healthcare recipient education:
  - Online education.
  - Written brochure/pamphlet.

5.2 HEALTHCARE WORKER STANDARDS
5.2.1 Establish and maintain competence
Implementing Standard 5.2.1

- Develop a system that makes safe employee behavior a key component in employee evaluations:
  - Annual competency attendance.
  - Participation in unit-/discipline-specific training.
- Serve as a role model for safe behavior.

5.2.2 Engage and educate the healthcare recipient regarding SPHM
Implementing Standard 5.2.2

- Provide feedback on written/electronic SPHM education tools pertaining to the healthcare recipient's understanding.
- Engage reluctant healthcare recipients by demonstrating technology.
- Develop confidence in using appropriate technology.
- Educate the family and/or caregiver on the need and how to use the Standards, especially across the care continuum into the home; this empowers the healthcare recipient and family to know what they need and ask for it.

Considerations for Community Settings: Employer–Vendor Resources

Healthcare workers employed in community settings such as home health agencies, assisted living facilities, or schools may encounter a wide variety of SPHM technology. When new SPHM technology will be used, training should be provided at the point of care, and the employer must ensure that the healthcare worker has access to a subject-matter expert for questions or consultation. Vendor-based written instructions for use, maintenance, and cleaning of technology are in place to assist workers in taking full advantage of technology. Periodic orientations with SPHM technology vendors or a local durable medical goods vendor may be helpful, and would provide a time for evaluative feedback on the special needs of community settings.

Evidence for Standard 5: Some Resources and Readings

American Nurses Association. (2013). *Safe patient handling and mobility: Interprofessional national standards.* Silver Spring, MD: Nursesbooks.org.

Cohen, M. A., Green, D. A., Nelson, G. G., Leib, R., Matz, M. A., et al. (2010). *Patient handling and movement assessments: A white paper* (Prepared by the 2010 Health Guidelines Revision Committee Specialty Subcommittee on Patient Movement). Dallas, TX: Facility Guidelines Institute. Retrieved August 7, 2013, from http://www.fgiguidelines.org/pdfs/FGI_PHAMA_whitepaper_042810.pdf

Committee on Quality of Healthcare in America, Institute of Medicine. (2001). *Crossing the quality chasm: A new health system for the 21st century.* Washington, DC: National Academies Press.

Dolan, P., Luo, J., Pollintine, P., Landham, P. R., Stefanakis, M., & Adams, M. A. (2013). Intervertebral disc decompression following endplate damage: Implications for disc degeneration depend on spinal level and age. Retrieved July 22, 2013, from http://www.ncbi.nlm.nih.gov/pubmed/23486408

Gaba, D. (2001). Structural and organizational issues in patient safety: A comparison of healthcare to other high-hazard industries. *California Management Review, 43,* 83–102.

Gaba, D. (2007). The future vision of simulation in healthcare. Simulation in Healthcare, 2, 126-135.

Gallagher, S. M. (2012). Intergenerational considerations in sustaining safe patient handling and mobility success: Implications in equipment usage. *American Journal of SPHM, 2*(4), 134-137.

Kohn, L., Corrigan, J., & Donaldson, M. (1999). To err is human: Building a safer health system. Washington, DC: National Academy Press.

Mohr, J., & Batalden, P. B. (2002). Improving safety on the front lines: The role of clinical microsystems. *Quality & Safety in Healthcare, 11*, 45–50.

Marras, W. (2008). *The trade-off in spine loads during patient pushing and pulling.* Geoff Kelafant Lecture (plenary address), 8th Annual Patient Handling and Movement Conference, Orlando, FL, March 12, 2008. Retrieved August 26, 2013, from http://ise.osu.edu/ISEFaculty/marras/marras.htm#2000

Moore, R. J. (2006). The vertebral endplate: Disc degeneration, disc regeneration. *European Spine Journal 15*(Suppl. 3), 333-337.

Nelson, A., Harwood, K. J., Tracey, C. A., & Dunn, K.L. (2008). Myths and facts about safe patient handling in rehabilitation. *Rehabilitation Nursing, 33*(1), 10-17. Retrieved August 26, 2013, from http://www.rehabnurse.org/uploads/files/pdf/sphchptr3.pdf

Nelson, E. C., Batalden, P. B., Huber, T. P., et al. (2002). Microsystems in healthcare. Part 1. Learning from high-performing front-line clinical units. *Joint Commission Journal of Quality Improvement, 28*, 472–493.

Ortiza, A. O., & Bordiaa, R. (2011). Injury to the vertebral endplate-disk complex associated with osteoporotic vertebral compression fractures. *AJNR, 32*, 115-120.

Schoenfisch, A. L., Pompeii, L. A., Myers, D. J., James, T., Yeung, Y., Fricklas, E., Pentico, M., & Lipscomb, H. J. (2011). Objective measures of adoption of patient lift and transfer devices to reduce nursing staff injuries in the hospital setting. *American Journal of Industrial Medicine, 54*(12), 935-945.

Staff at Mayo Clinic (2012). Weight training dos and don'ts. Retrieved July 21, 2013, from http://www.mayoclinic.com/health/weight-training/SM00028/NSECTIONGROUP=2

Waters, T. R. (1999). Evaluation of the revised NIOSH lifting equation. *SPINE, 24*(4), 386-395.

Waters, T. R. (2011). Product design issues related to safe patient handling technology. In W. Karwowski, M. M. Soares, & N. A. Stanton (Eds.), *Human factors and ergonomics in consumer product design: Uses and applications* (pp. 89-100). Boca Raton, FL: CRC Press.

Standard 6. Integrated SPHM Assessment, Care Planning, and Technology Use

I've had two back surgeries and two knee surgeries from pushing gurneys on those carpeted halls. It destroyed my back and knees. I had vocational rehab and 6 months on-the-job training, I am in a very sedentary job, and have gained 25 pounds in 5 months.

Standard 6. Integrate Patient-Centered SPHM Assessment, Plan of Care, and Use of SPHM Technology

The employer and healthcare workers partner to adapt the plan of care to meet the SPHM needs of individual healthcare recipients and specify appropriate SPHM technology and methods.

Putting It All Together for Success

The Institute of Medicine (IOM) defines *patient-centered care* as "[p]roviding care that is respectful of and responsive to individual patient preferences, needs, and values, and ensuring that patient values guide all clinical decisions." Patient-centered health care is the healthcare system designed and delivered to address the healthcare needs and preferences of the healthcare recipient. The value of patient-centered care is that health care becomes more clinically appropriate and cost-effective. To that end, patient-centered health care supports active involvement of healthcare recipients and family members in the implementation of innovative care strategies, such as SPHM. Recognizing the healthcare recipient as a unique individual is essential to the next step, which is to integrate SPHM technology into the plan of care based on SPHM assessment.

Informing the healthcare recipient about the SPHM program is important. There are a number of ways to accomplish this. The best time to begin involving the healthcare recipient is at the time of admission or preadmission. Consider a written brochure that summarizes goals and expectations specific to the SPHM program. Christiana Hospital in Wilmington, Delaware, uses a specially designed pamphlet, which has been developed based on the learning needs of the healthcare recipient, family members, and visitors. The pamphlet is instructional for the healthcare recipient, serves as a guide for the healthcare worker who is describing the SPHM program at Christiana, and sets the tone for questions about the SPHM program (Price, 2012). Another strategy, which has been successful at Veterans Affairs (VA) facilities, is a continuous-loop video that plays on the televisions in the patients' rooms. This video, titled "Flying, Gliding and Sliding," provides a basic orientation to the SPHM program at the VA facilities as it describes lifts, slings, slides, lateral transfer devices, and other technology. Further, this presentation provides a mechanism to manage expectations, especially when the healthcare recipient has not had the experience of care at a minimal lift facility.

The Society of Hospital Medicine (n.d.) describes its "Mobility Assessment Test: Performance Based" as a mobility assessment tool that can be performed in less than one minute. This particular tool screens for gait and balance impairments. The performance-based mobility test is named "Timed—Get Up and GO!" The test is performed with the healthcare recipient wearing regular footwear, using a usual walking aid if needed, and sitting back in a chair with armrests. On the word "Go," the patient is asked to do the following: (1) stand up from the chair, (2) walk nine feet in one direction, (3) turn, (4) walk back to the chair, and (5) sit down. Scoring is related to the time needed to accomplish the task safely. If the task is performed in less than 10 seconds, findings are normal. A time of 20 seconds or more is an abnormal score. For example, low scores correlate with good functional independence; high scores correlate with poor functional independence and higher risk of falls and other hazards of immobility.

Banner Health has piloted a validated mobility assessment tool called the Bedside Mobility Assessment Tool (BMAT). This easy-to-use assessment tool is designed to predict mobility and then set criteria for SPHM needs, based on the assessment. The BMAT is integrated into the Banner electronic medical record system-wide. All registered nurses in the inpatient setting perform the mobility assessment every shift and as needed, assigning each patient a level of mobility.

Implementation Ideas and Insights for Standard 6

What follows are selected ideas and insights on implementing the SPHM standard on integrating a patient-centered approach that coordinates assessment, the plan of care, and supporting technology. Matching technology to the healthcare recipient's unique needs is key. A comprehensive mobility assessment is fundamental to selecting an appropriate plan of care; however, a written procedure that links the mobility status to SPHM technology is imperative to success. The ideas and insights are organized by the sets and subsets of the standards that are required by any facility: one specific to your organization as an employer, the other to your facility's interprofessional healthcare workers. Communication, delegation, and transitions of care are included as components of this standard.

6.1 EMPLOYER STANDARDS

6.1.1 Provide a written procedure on the SPHM assessment and plan of care

Implementing Standard 6.1.1

- Develop a written procedure on how to assess, evaluate, or score a healthcare recipient's needs; this should include a standardized tool for assessing mobility, cognition, and ability to participate in activities.
- Establish an algorithm or process to match healthcare recipient needs and goals with SPHM technology, such as the VA Safe Patient Handling and Movement Algorithms.

6.1.2 Require initial and ongoing assessment or process to determine SPHM needs

Implementing Standard 6.1.2

- Develop a procedure to assess a healthcare recipient's SPHM needs that affect immobility:
  - Determine a frequency for ongoing assessment based on research findings and organization-specific risk and injury data.
  - Include provisions for physical, cognitive, clinical, and rehabilitative needs, such as those included in the VA *Safe Patient Handling Guidebook*.
  - Establish a method for communicating and documenting assessment findings, such as documentation consistent with ANA's Principles for Nursing Documentation, which may be adapted to interdisciplinary documentation.

6.1.3 Include SPHM in the plan of care

Implementing Standard 6.1.3

- Establish a process to link the individual plan of care to SPHM technology and methods such as a clinical pathway or map, which incorporates mobility assessment findings, task to accomplish, and technology and worker(s) to support the task, as well as a timeline to achieve certain mobility goals.
- Identify a strategy to link the individual plan of care to expected outcomes:
  - Incorporate data collection into the documentation process, such as with a mobility assessment indicator (e.g., minimal, moderate, maximum), the Braden Score for Assessment of Pressure Sore Risk, or the Morse Fall Scale.
  - Establish a method to analyze collected data, recognizing that risk management, quality improvement, occupational health, and other departments are continuously collecting this data; it is then a function of identifying the point of contact for the data and coordinating distribution of the data.
  - Communicate outcome data that have been collected and analyzed to end users and managers, as a way to begin to determine whether individual care plans (along with required technology) are meeting the expected outcomes. Communication of outcome data may be accomplished through unit-based reports, unit-based meetings, or individual verbal communication.
  - Manage outcomes as necessary for ongoing success, such as activities described in Standard 8.1, wherein outcome management is described as a method to meaningfully link behaviors to outcomes.
- Include mobility assessment in each plan of care.
- Include the healthcare recipient, family members, and visitors in order to better manage expectations associated with use of technology and worker support.
- Recognize mobility as a strategy to return to baseline, an approach consistent with early, progressive mobility practices.

6.1.4 Address SPHM at transitions of care

Implementing Standard 6.1.4

- Develop a written communication tool to address SPHM at transitions of care (discharge plan):
  - Consider integrating communication processes into existing communication tools.

- Identify use of specific SPHM technology.
- Indicate the response of the healthcare recipient to SPHM technology.
■ Integrate SPHM information/resources into handoff communication:
  - Develop a policy/procedure to incorporate SPHM information and resources, including the specific technology the healthcare recipient has used and assessment scores, such as mobility scale (e.g., BMAT), pressure ulcer risk (e.g., Braden Scale for Pressure Ulcer Risk), or physical and cognitive abilities (Functional Independence Measure [FIM]).
  - Provide processes, such as steps to handoff communication, either verbally, electronically, or in hard-copy form.
  - Integrate SPHM information/resources into any handoff documentation and include it in electronic records.
  - Ensure training that includes SPHM information/resources.

6.1.5 Provide a system to resolve healthcare recipient's refusal
Implementing Standard 6.1.5

■ Recognize the value of the risk manager, hospital attorney, and patient service/advocate as individuals who fully understand the liability and risk associated with failure to provide safe care to the healthcare recipient because of the recipient's refusal to accept SPHM technology.

■ Develop a policy to address healthcare recipient refusal, but keep in mind that a clear explanation delivered in a standard and acceptable format is a strategy for communicating safe handling and mobility expectation with the healthcare recipient; nevertheless, a policy to address healthcare recipient refusal will include a chain of command to address the issue, as well as identifying (by title) resources who should have input into the refusal and can make themselves available to address the worker's concerns.

■ Include a unit-specific procedure for healthcare recipient refusal which is similar to (and congruent with) the facility-wide policy, but incorporates the specific concerns of the unit or practice area.

■ Reinforce strategies to address healthcare recipient refusal as part of education/training, such as communication skills and methods to approach introduction of equipment (including determining why the refusal has occurred; for example, does the worker seem to lack confidence in use of the technology? Should the lift coach or champion introduce technology if the worker initially lacks confidence, or is there another solution that would better serves the safety of the healthcare worker and recipient?).

- Review use of electronic/written tools to present the SPHM program, in a manner that supports the learning needs of the healthcare recipient, family members, or visitors.
- Provide unit- or discipline-specific training to establish confidence in technology use, whether training includes actual use of the equipment or a method to access resources to serve as champion or coach.

6.1.6 Monitor healthcare recipient injuries associated with patient handling and mobility
Implementing Standard 6.1.6

- Recognize the value of the organization's risk management and quality improvement services; these departments, regardless of practice setting, have access to data on healthcare recipient injuries associated with patient handling and mobility and generally embrace opportunities to improve costly outcomes.
- Recognize the value of the organization's clinical experts, which is determined by the practice setting. Experts could include, for example (but are not limited to) the wound care nurse in home care to monitor pressure ulcer outcomes, a critical care clinician to monitor incidence of ICU-acquired pneumonia, or a corporate safety officer in an assisted living setting to monitor worker injuries.
- Collect data pertaining to healthcare recipient safety outcome indicators such NDNQI®. OSHA 300 logs aligned with reports from worker's compensation data help tell a story that may reveal an association between injured workers and injuries sustained by healthcare recipients. This is one method of making the business case for the facility:
  - Hospital-acquired pressure ulcers:
    - Frequency.
    - Severity.
  - Fall-related injuries.
  - Pneumonia.
  - Hospital-acquired urinary tract infections.
  - Healthcare recipient satisfaction.
- Establish a process to quantify costs of healthcare recipient injuries over time:
  - Determine frequency of data analysis.
  - Communicate data to stakeholders.
  - Manage risk/adverse outcomes based on data.

6.1.7 Support safe delegation of SPHM tasks and activities

Implementing Standard 6.1.7

■ Evaluate delegation of SPHM tasks and activities as to whether they are in keeping with the healthcare worker's training, experience, education, and license.

■ Recognize state practice acts.

■ Recognize legislation governing licensure.

■ Recognize specific regulations pertaining to unlicensed personnel.

■ Recognize SPHM legislation (state/national) pertaining to tasks and activities.

6.2 HEALTHCARE WORKER STANDARDS

6.2.1 Perform initial and ongoing assessment of mobility and SPHM needs

Implementing Standard 6.2.1

■ Determine whether a mobility and/or needs assessment tool is available for use.

■ If assessment tools are unavailable, develop a tool based on PHAMA (Cohen et al., 2010) and other resources:

● Perform an initial assessment and communicate findings (medical record as indicated).

● Perform ongoing assessments per policy or as indicated based on professional judgment.

6.2.2 Communicate with the healthcare recipient and family

Implementing Standard 6.2.2

■ Recognize the value of marketing, patient care services, clinical departments, customer relations, end users, and others who create a meaningful standard and organization-wide story to share with the healthcare recipient and family members.

■ Provide written or electronic information pertaining to the SPHM program, its purpose, and its safety goals:

● Include family members and visitors as appropriate to manage expectations concerning use of the technology, and the fact that use of technology will change as the assessments indicate changes in mobility.

● Establish understanding as evidenced by appropriate questions and verbal attestation of understanding.

● Document the healthcare recipient's response to training, such as the degree of understanding and expectations when appropriate.

6.2.3 Address SPHM at transitions of care
Implementing Standard 6.2.3
- Provide information pertaining to SPHM technology or necessary tasks/ skills or assessment scores at transitions of care:
  - Provide written information per facility policy.
  - Provide verbal communication per facility policy.
- Include the SPHM plan of care in discharge planning; this can be accomplished using the hard-copy or electronic discharge planning form or other communication document.
- Include the SPHM plan of care at each transition of care, such as from long-term care to home care, from special education to the public school setting, or from home care to an assisted living facility; this can be accomplished electronically, via the medical record or other communication document.

6.2.4 Delegate care tasks in a safe manner
Implementing Standard 6.2.4
- Identify state professional practice acts or other applicable laws or regulations pertaining to delegation or assignment of tasks. Professional practice acts can be found electronically, or the risk manager or compliance officer may provide guidance as to applicable laws or regulations. Unions representing healthcare workers are often very well informed on these statutes and are forthcoming with this information, and the organization or health system's attorneys can be valuable partners if resources allow.
- Identify job descriptions, policies, or procedures of the organization that pertain to delegation or assignment of tasks.

Considerations for Community Settings: Assisted Living Facility
The assisted living setting is a rapidly growing sector, with an estimated 1 million American seniors choosing this living environment. Further, there are approximately 77 million "baby boomers" planning retirement in the next two decades.

Sara was an 84-year-old, completely independent woman who entered assisted living because of her late husband's physical limitations. When her husband passed, she realized she had made many friends and enjoyed the staff members and the physical layout of the environment, and therefore decided to stay. Yesterday, Sara tripped and twisted her knee. Today, she is having trouble walking, standing, and even getting out of bed safely. Sara's healthcare providers believe these limitations are temporary; however, the concern is that a transfer to a nursing home for additional assistance may be unnecessarily detrimental, both emotionally and physically, to this otherwise independent woman. Safety technology such as walkers, sit-to-stand, or even a mechanical lift-bed can facilitate mobility and independence in such cases. Opportunities are expanding for the healthcare worker to provide information on appropriate and available SPHM technologies and supplies, matching the resident's limitation to resources that are available—either short or long term. Healthcare recipients and their families must be central to the process of selection. Helping the family and resident understand the importance of the SPHM technology is critical in obtaining their buy-in. The use of SPHM technology in long-term care, and specifically in assisted living settings, is an important part of promoting independence. A progression through different technologies may indicate a functional change: possibly deterioration, possibly improvement.

Evidence for Standard 6: Some Resources and Readings

American Nurses Association. (2103). *Safe patient handling and mobility: Interprofessional national standards.* Silver Spring, MD: Nursesbooks.org.

Berwick, D. (2009). What patient-centered should mean: Confessions of an extremist. *Health Affairs Web Exclusive.* Retrieved May 22, 2013, from http:// content.healthaffairs.org/content/28/4/w555.abstract

Cohen, M. A., Green, D. A., Nelson, G. G., Leib, R., Matz, M. A., et al. (2010). *Patient handling and movement assessments: A white paper* (Prepared by the 2010 Health Guidelines Revision Committee Specialty Subcommittee on Patient Movement). Dallas, TX: Facility Guidelines Institute. Retrieved August 7, 2013, from http://www.fgiguidelines.org/pdfs/FGI_PHAMA_whitepaper_042810.pdf

Gill, P. S. (2013). Improving health outcomes: Applying dimensions of employee engagement to patients. *International Journal of Health, Wellness & Society, 3*(1), 1-9.

Gill, P. S. (2013). Patient engagement: An investigation at a primary care clinic. *International Journal of General Medicine, 6,* 85–98.

Institute for Healthcare Improvement. *Patient centered care.* Retrieved May 21, 2013, from http://www.ihi.org/IHI/Topics/PatientCenteredCare/ PatientCenteredCareGeneral/

Institute on Medicine. *Crossing the quality chasm: A new health system for the 21st century.* Retrieved June 22, 2013, from http://iom.edu/Reports/2001/Crossing-the-Quality-Chasm-A-New-Health-System-for-the-21st-Century.aspx

Mathias, S., Nayak, U. S. L., & Isaacs, B. (1986). Balance in elderly patients: "The
Get Up and Go" test. *Archives of Physical Medicine & Rehabilitation, 67,*
387-389.

Podsiadlo, D., & Richardson, S. (1991). The timed "Up and Go": A test of basic
functional mobility for frail elderly persons. *Journal of the American Geriatrics
Society, 39,* 142-148.

Price, C. (2012). Personal communication/conversation with author, November 8,
2012.

Safe Patient Handling and Movement. Algorithms. In *Safe patient handling
guidebook.* Retrieved July 29, 2013, from www.visn8.va.gov

Society of Hospital Medicine. (n.d.). Mobility assessment test: Performance based.
(Clinical Tool Box for Geriatric Care). Retrieved August 26, 2013, from http://
www.hospitalmedicine.org/geriresource/toolbox/mobility_assessment_tools.htm

Zaine, E. E. (2012). Joint Commission Center for Transforming Healthcare releases
tool to tackle miscommunication among caregivers. Retrieved May 29, 2013,
from http://www.jointcommission.org/center_transforming_healthcare_tst_hoc/

Standard 7. SPHM in Reasonable Accommodation and Post-Injury Return to Work

I have an urge to paint an abstract that depicts how it feels to be injured and disgraced by the employer. Lots of red....

Standard 7. Include SPHM in Reasonable Accommodation and Post-Injury Return to Work

The employer and healthcare workers partner to establish a comprehensive SPHM program that can help the employer provide reasonable accommodations to healthcare workers who were injured.

Bridging a Partnership with Employers and Healthcare Workers

Although most SPHM programs include technology, policies and procedures, and training, many programs fail to recognize the value of integrating ways health-care workers can join their efforts with those of employers to develop a strategy for reasonable accommodation in the presence of injury. Eric Race, founder and CEO of Atlas Lift Tech, explains that occupational health coordinators are embracing SPHM efforts because they now are confident they are releasing post-injury workers into a safe working environment (Race, 2013). One of the most important factors in recovering from an occupational injury and controlling worker's compensation costs is facilitation of a meaningful and safe return to work effort. The healthcare worker benefits by being productive and receiving a salary, and the employer benefits by having an experienced healthcare worker back on the job. However, a safe return to work environment is essential.

Planning for healthcare worker recovery and return to work is an important component of a SPHM program. A first step for such an action plan is acknowledging the value of a partnership between the employer and the healthcare worker. Consider Madge, a 32-year-old nursing assistant who had worked at the same home care agency for the past 17 years. Madge had always manually handled healthcare recipients at home. While Madge was away with her shoulder injury, the agency instituted an organization-wide SPHM program that coincided with the programs at the local acute and long-term care facilities. As part of the program, Madge was trained on the principles of SPHM before she was released back to work. She served as a champion for the SPHM program.

Healthcare workers such as Madge need appropriate medical care/intervention and a safe return to work. If the provider restricts the work the healthcare worker can perform, the healthcare worker can expect to be assigned modified or alternate work duties designed to facilitate a return to work. *Modified work* is often described as the injured healthcare worker's regular job that is modified to accommodate work restrictions. *Alternative work* is considered to be a temporary work assignment when the worker is unable to return to his or her regular job. Transitional work should be work that the healthcare worker can perform with an acceptable degree of efficiency without endangering his or her health and safety or that of others. *Transitional work* allows an injured healthcare worker to remain safely in the workplace, but in a modified or alternate work capacity until she or he has recovered sufficiently to return to her or his regular job.

For this partnership to work, employers and healthcare workers must take on certain responsibilities. This is especially true in occupational settings where workers, historically, have been expected to manually lift, turn, and reposition healthcare recipients numerous times throughout the workday. Recognizing SPHM in both reasonable accommodation and the post-injury return to work is a key factor in this partnership.

Implementation Ideas and Insights for Standard 7

What follows are selected ideas and insights on strategies to include reasonable accommodation and post-injury return to work processes into a meaningful SPHM program. A collaborative approach to managing the challenge of injury is essential. Ways to create a mutually respectful environment evolve from the partnership that is built between the healthcare worker and the employer. Understanding and managing occupational hazards through thorough ergonomic assessments tailored to the special needs of injured workers is part of the process. The ideas and insights are organized by the sets and subsets of the standards that are required by any facility: one specific to your organization as an employer, the other to your facility's interprofessional healthcare workers. This approach recognizes teamwork as a factor inherent in a successful, safe, and healthy occupational environment that addresses the goals of the healthcare worker, healthcare recipient, and healthcare organization.

7.1 EMPLOYER STANDARDS

7.1.1 Facilitate the employment of disabled workers

Implementing Standard 7.1.1

- Establish a method to evaluate any physical limitations of the healthcare worker, and ensure that the method is compliant with the Americans with Disabilities Act.
- Identify the range of physical demands of the job, such as pushing, pulling, and lifting up to 35 pounds of static weight.
- Establish a process to match an injured healthcare worker to the physical demands of the job:
  - Provide ergonomic analysis that is compliant with the Americans with Disabilities Act.
  - Review SPHM technology, such as floor- or ceiling-based lifts, a variety of slings, lateral transfer devices, and/or sit-to-stand technology.
  - Train employees in SPHM skills such as sling selection, selection of appropriate transfer devices, and use of full-body lateral rotation air support as an adjunct for turning (not repositioning, which still must be done manually).

7.1.2 Monitor healthcare worker injuries associated with patient handling and mobility

Implementing Standard 7.1.2

- Recognize that a standard, accepted format for recording occupational injuries is in place, in the form of OSHA 300 logs in conjunction with worker's compensation data for identification of occupational injuries associated with patient handling. This includes frequency and severity of injuries and costs over time per injury.
- Identify, by title, the individual within the organization who manages worker injury data associated with lifting, transfers, repositioning, or mobility; even slips, trips, and falls may count if related to patient handling.

- Collect baseline data on injuries:
  - Frequency.
  - Severity.
  - Cost.
- Analyze data for purposes of meaningful injury management once the SPHM is in place:
  - Assess frequency, which may increase because of awareness pertaining to reporting and early intervention.
  - Reduce severity.
  - Reduce cost, recognizing that even though frequency of injuries is likely to increase, severity and therefore costs can be expected to decrease.

7.1.3 Facilitate early return to work following injury
Implementing Standard 7.1.3

- Recognize the value of the human resources, employee health, occupational medicine, and patient care services, as these departments are both involved and interested in safe and early return to work strategies.
- Establish, implement, and sustain a process to help injured healthcare workers to return to work as quickly as possible:
  - Identify ergonomic opportunities (see Standard 7.1.1).
  - Recognize medical restrictions.

7.2 HEALTHCARE WORKER STANDARDS
7.2.1 Notify the employer of physical limitations or restrictions
Implementing Standard 7.2.1

- Identify facility-specific policies for notifying the employer of any physical limitations.
- Provide up-to-date medical documentation:
  - Identify any physical limitations, such as lifting limits, fatigue, or discomfort.
  - Identify occupational restrictions such as cognitive abilities or lifting limits.

7.2.2 Participate in the return to work plan
Implementing Standard 7.2.2

- Request reasonable accommodation from the employer if necessary.
- Report any further injuries promptly.
- Stay in contact with healthcare providers.

- Attend all medical treatment appointments.
- Follow medical restrictions both on and off the job.
- Accept transitional work (modified or alternate work duties) as provided by the employer if you are unable to return to your pre-injury job.

Considerations for Community Settings: Rural Long-Term Care Settings

Every healthcare organization must have a system for evaluating, managing, and reducing healthcare worker injuries, with the goal of building a partnership for safety. Consider Angelina, a nurse's assistant at a 49-bed long-term care facility in a rural community, who explains that most of her workers complain of back pain much of time. Angelina reports that the turnover is so high that by the time her co-workers are trained in use of the lift, they generally move on to a different job. A significant amount of manual lifting and moving takes place. Early state legislation and resolutions addressed nurses in acute general hospitals. Certainly this population is important; however, these mandates discount injuries among all healthcare workers in a number of subacute settings, including long-term care. To ensure a healthy pool of healthcare workers across practice settings, it is imperative to consider reasonable accommodation and post-injury return to work programs as part of SPHM across the transitions in care.

Evidence for Standard 7: Some Resources and Readings

American Nurses Association. (2103). *Safe patient handling and mobility: Interprofessional national standards.* Silver Spring, MD: Nursesbooks.org.

Centers for Disease Control. (2013). *NIOSH workplace safety and health topics: Safe patient handling.* Retrieved May 21, 2013, from http://www.cdc.gov/niosh/topics/safepatient/

Cohen, M. A., Green, D. A., Nelson, G. G., Leib, R., Matz, M. A., et al. (2010). *Patient handling and movement assessments: A white paper* (Prepared by the 2010 Health Guidelines Revision Committee Specialty Subcommittee on Patient Movement). Dallas, TX: Facility Guidelines Institute. Retrieved August 7, 2013, from http://www.fgiguidelines.org/pdfs/FGI_PHAMA_whitepaper_042810.pdf

Collins, J. W., Bell, J. L., & Gronqvist, R. (2010). Developing evidence-based interventions to address the leading causes of workers' compensation among healthcare workers. *Rehabilitation Nursing, 35*(6), 225-235, 261.

Job Accommodation Network. (2013). *Occupation and industry series: Accommodating nurses with disabilities.* Retrieved July 29, 2013, from http://askjan.org/media/nurses.html

Mattei, S. Y. (2012, June). *A report to New Yorkers: The case for caring technology.* New York, NY: New Yorkers for Patient & Family Empowerment. Retrieved June 22, 2013, from http://patientandfamily.org/

Race, E. (2013). Personal communication with author.

U.S. Equal Employment Opportunity Commission. (2011). *Questions and answers about health care workers and the Americans with Disabilities Act.* Retrieved June 3, 2013, from http://www.eeoc.gov/facts/health_care_workers.html

Standard 8. Comprehensive SPHM Evaluation Program

They make lift equipment, but the hospital doesn't want it. They say it costs too much.

Standard 8. Establish a Comprehensive Evaluation System

The employer and healthcare workers partner to establish a comprehensive system to evaluate SPHM program status, using staff performance, staff injury incidence and severity, and healthcare recipient outcome metrics.

Crafting a Database to Tell a Compelling Story

The development and availability of standards for patient safety can serve several purposes. Standards establish minimum levels of performance, establish consistency or uniformity across disciplines and practice settings, and promote reproducible outcomes. Another purpose of standards is to set expectations for healthcare recipients and healthcare workers. Standards can be used in public regulatory processes, such as licensure for health professionals and healthcare organizations, such as hospitals or health plans. However, compliance with professional standards such as the *ANA Safe Patient Handling and Mobility Interprofessional National Standards* is entirely voluntary.

Although there are many kinds of standards in health care, few standards focus explicitly on issues of patient safety. Further, even fewer provisions are made to evaluate the comprehensive nature of a SPHM program. To evaluate the clinical and economic performance of a SPHM program, a process must be in place to collect complex data and provide a method of communicating the data in a straightforward manner. For example, under one safety-based program, trained healthcare workers used mechanical lifts and repositioning devices rather than manual lifts and handling. In this particular case, researchers identified a 49% reduction in patient falls related to lift and transfer activities (Mattei, 2012). Proponents of this program also indicated that mechanical lift techniques free healthcare workers from the burden of lifting patients so they can devote their energies to direct patient care activities.

A robust process that generates reports on program indicators, both clinically and economically, helps the champions of the SPHM program meet goals and identify opportunities for improvement. However, it is essential that nursing not shoulder the actual work of the evaluation process. The goal of a successful SPHM team is to establish a process wherein data is provided by those in the organization who already have a mechanism in place for data collection; those data are analyzed at the point of extraction by stakeholders who are aware of their responsibilities to the SPHM team, which includes providing annotated information to the SPHM team for synthesis, evaluation, and publication.

New or emerging SPHM programs best serve their long-term objectives by recognizing opportunities for measurement early in the effort, which is the purpose of the tool titled, "Who can get me what I want?" which is the first step to a business case. (See the introduction.) This provides a reasonable baseline from which to measure and later manage. Mature programs, which have used worker's compensation data as the sole means of gauging success, may find that use of more complex data is a meaningful way to demonstrate the value of sustaining SPHM investments over time. For instance, the Celano model (see the introduction) can be used over time to continue to support the business case for an evolving program. Ongoing improvement efforts, from quality, cost, and risk perspectives, are best managed by recognizing success and failures, and using recognized deficiencies as opportunities to further transform the SPHM program into a culture of safety.

Implementation Ideas and Insights for Standard 8

What follows are selected ideas and insights on implementing the SPHM standard on establishing a comprehensive evaluation system. The direct and indirect impact and value of SPHM is just now coming into focus. For example, in 2008 a hospital in the northeastern United States created an early ICU rehab program with dedicated physical and occupational therapists, which added about $358,000 to the cost of care annually. However, by 2009, the length of stay in the MICU had decreased an average of 23%, down from 6.5 days to 5 days, while the time spent by those same patients as they transitioned to less-intensive hospital units within the hospital fell 18% as compared with those not participating in the ICU rehab program. Using a financial model, the estimated net cost saving for the hospital was about $818,000 per year, even after factoring in the up-front costs. This program, framed within the context of a SPHM program, has the potential to capture a variety of positive outcomes associated with improved mobility status across units within the facility and may impact readmission outcomes and functional status in the post-acute care areas (American Physical Therapy Association [APTA], 2013).

The ideas and insights described herein are organized by the sets and subsets of the standards that are required by any facility: one specific to your organization as an employer, the other to your facility's interprofessional health-care worker. Collecting and managing evidence by way of a comprehensive evaluation system drives longevity and sustainability of the SPHM program over time, by demonstrating return on investment from the perspective of the healthcare recipient and worker.

8.1 EMPLOYER STANDARDS

8.1.1 Establish a comprehensive evaluation system

Implementing Standard 8.1.1

- Ensure quality/performance improvement during planning phases (see Standard 1.1.1):
  - Ensure that SPHM goals and objectives align with other safety initiatives of the organization. For example, consider early progressive mobility initiatives that serve the long- and short-term patient quality indicators; without a SPHM culture of safety, this practice can be a threat to worker safety. Or consider a new customer service initiative at the outpatient center which includes free valet parking—but employees are asked to assist visitors and healthcare recipients from their vehicles without mechanical technology or training, which poses a threat to worker safety.
- Recognize the interdisciplinary evolution/maturity of the SPHM program.
- Recognize the value of ongoing measurement activities. These measurement activities will be as unique as the organization, unit, discipline, and individual worker. Metrics ought to align with data, as described in Standards 2.1.1 and 8.1.3:
  - Systems/organizational performance may be measured (for example, by determining if slide sheets are available in adequate quantities for safe in-bed positioning based on collected data that describe the numbers of in-bed positioning tasks over a designated period of time).

- Unit- and discipline-based performance may be measured (for example, by investigating the time to mobility in a critical care unit among a certain kind of healthcare recipients).
- In the state of California, for example, healthcare worker performance may be measured by determining the numbers of healthcare workers who have learned the Five Areas of Exposure as defined by CA AB 1136, along with technology to address the care task in the area of exposure.

8.1.2 Identify a variety of data sources and measures
Implementing Standard 8.1.2

- Assemble an interdisciplinary team (see Standard 2.1.1).
- Identify appropriate quality indicators for measurement (see Standards 2.1.2 and 8.1.3):
  - Perform a literature search to identify appropriate quality indicators, such as fall-related injuries, pressure ulcer development, catheter-related urinary tract infections, or satisfaction among healthcare workers or recipients:
    - Unit-specific, such as falls during toileting because of failure to accommodate elderly, weak healthcare recipients who believe they are capable of ambulating independently to the bathroom.
    - Discipline-specific, such as a healthcare recipient who becomes combative during manual handling when a therapist attempts strengthening activities.
    - Facility-specific, such as poor communication about the process for laundering and storing slings.
- Identify, by title, the individual most closely aligned with/accountable for management of quality indicators (see the introduction for "Who can get me what I want?"):
  - Identify the most standardized, widely accepted tool for measuring the quality indicator.
  - Identify standard definitions and terms pertaining to the quality indicator.
- Establish a data collection, analysis, and reporting mechanism, such as NDNQI® and others, if such a mechanism is not already in place.

8.1.3 Utilize evidence-based methods for data collection and analysis
Implementing Standard 8.1.3

- Identify, by title, the individual(s) most closely aligned with/accountable for management of quality indicators (see Standard 8.1.2).

- Obtain baseline data on as many quality indicators as possible; however, in the early stages of the SPHM program development, consider identifying a limited number of healthcare recipient safety indicators to study. The limited number of quality indicators should be decided by seeking high-cost, high-frequency, high-risk indicators; once identified, this limited number of indicators should be measured very frequently (e.g., quarterly) and reported frequently. There should also be a method to sustain interest and enthusiasm in the program by creating and publicizing some early and meaningful wins.

  - Healthcare worker safety data primarily become available by analyzing OSHA 300 logs and worker's compensation claims to establish the injury costs specific to patient handling; these data are available from the risk management department or its designee:
    - Incidence of MSD.
    - Severity of MSD.
    - Costs of MSD.
    - Number of light/modified/restricted duty days due to handling injuries.
    - Number of lost workdays due to handling injuries.
    - Prevalence of musculoskeletal discomfort in healthcare workers may be evaluated using an anonymous survey tool or by interviewing workers.

  - Healthcare recipient safety is monitored by the risk management and or quality improvement departments using universally appropriate measurement tools as mandated by NDNQI®, The Joint Commission, the state department of health, and others. It is important that the data be collected, monitored, reported, and available for purposes such as associating the SPHM program with the following quality indicators:
    - Adverse patient event: fall-related injuries.
    - Adverse patient event: DVT/PE.
    - Adverse patient event: pneumonia.
    - Adverse patient event: HAPU.
    - Frequency with which healthcare workers are able to mobilize patients.
    - Readmission within 30 days.

  - Other:
    - Healthcare worker recruitment and retention.
    - Satisfaction on the part of the healthcare worker and recipient.
    - Community awareness and support.

8.1.4 Disseminate findings
Implementing Standard 8.1.4

- Identify existing methods within the organization for disseminating findings pertaining to other initiatives, such as monthly unit meetings, annual state-of-the-organization presentations, and intranet communication boards.
- Identify creative, interesting methods to communicate findings:
  - Provide electronic summaries of data.
  - Develop attractive printed materials:
    - Flyers.
    - Posters.
    - Other.
- Utilize group meetings to discuss/present SPHM findings:
  - Include healthcare workers.
  - Include the management team.
  - Include the leadership team.
  - Include community members when appropriate.
- Focus on success:
  - Feature an individual (a healthcare worker) when appropriate.
  - Feature processes when appropriate.
  - Feature unit- or discipline-specific successes.

8.1.5 Develop a plan for quality improvement and remediation of deficiencies
Implementing Standard 8.1.5

A diverse group of stakeholders (see Standard 2.1.1) will review the data and develop recommendations. The organization will develop and implement a plan or activities to remediate deficiencies within a reasonable time.

- Assemble a peer-review, interdisciplinary team:
  - Quality/performance improvement.
  - Risk management.
  - Patient care services:
    - Therapy.
    - Nursing.
    - Medicine.
  - Others.
- Review opportunities for improvement, such as near misses, adverse outcomes, decreases in satisfaction, or increases in severity or costs of injury.
- Identify appropriate opportunities for improvement.

- Examine why deficiencies exist:
  - Is administrative support in place and visible?
  - Is a systems deficiency identified?
  - Are healthcare workers held accountable in the SPHM initiative?
  - Is a process for change management in place?
  - Do quality indicators accurately assess process and structure outcomes?
  - Is there another explanation for deficiencies?
- Develop recommendations.
- Implement an action plan.
- Create provisions to measure outcomes.

8.1.6 Comply with the organization's policies, professional codes of ethics, privacy laws and regulations, and other regulatory language

Implementing Standard 8.1.6

- Recognize the value of the corporate compliance department, risk management, quality/performance improvement, legal team members, facility leadership, and others in complying with policies, regulations, and more.
- Review the SPHM program for compliance with existing organizational policies, appropriate professional codes of ethics, the Health Insurance Portability Privacy and Accountability Act, the Americans with Disabilities Act, state worker's compensation laws, and other applicable codes and regulations.

8.2 HEALTHCARE WORKER STANDARDS

8.2.1 Assist with data collection

Implementing Standard 8.2.1

- Participate in data collection when possible, and provide accurate information during the data collection process.
- Participate in communication activities:
  - Seek unit-specific opportunities.
  - Seek discipline-specific opportunities.

8.2.2 Comply with the organization's policies, professional codes of ethics, privacy laws and regulations, and other regulatory language

Implementing Standard 8.2.2

- Identify organizational policies:
  - Review and integrate general policies into practice.

- Review and integrate SPHM policies, procedures, algorithms, and guide-lines into practice.
- Identify professional codes of ethics:
  - Comply with state and federal regulations.
  - Provide personal privacy:
    - Healthcare worker.
    - Healthcare recipient.
- Comply with discipline-specific codes of ethics and practice acts.

Considerations for Community Settings: Research Opportunities in the Long-Term Care Setting

Quality indicators have been driving evidence-based care in acute care settings for at least the past two decades. As trends toward accountable care organizations and increased numbers of healthcare recipients receiving care in the subacute care settings increase, the value of practices that follow the evidence will gain momentum across all continuums of care. Every healthcare organization must have a system in place for evaluating and improving the effectiveness of its SPHM program by way of a comprehensive evaluation system. This is especially true in long-term care settings: There the rate of lost-time sprains and strains in private nursing homes is more than three times the national average, and for back injuries it is almost four times the national average. To that end, in 2009 a study conducted in the state of Ohio demonstrated that a $500 technology purchase per nursing home worker was associated with a 21% reduction in the back injury rate (D'Arcy, Sasai, & Stearns, 2012). These authors explained that regions without widespread access to lifting devices may be able to reduce injury rates by increasing the availability of lifting devices, and that the potential for reductions in injury rates in the United States is most enhanced by improving training and ensuring adequate time for resident care, as most facilities currently have lifts available. Further, consider research designed to investigate factors that contribute to injury among nursing assistants in the long-term care/nursing home setting. The same Ohio study suggested that lack of training, high turnover rates, and poor staffing levels were associated with injuries (D'Arcy, Sasai, & Stearns, 2012). Of interest were the inconsistent findings pertaining to acuity. The authors suggested that facilities that accepted healthcare recipients with a higher acuity were more likely to include lifting technology in the plan of care, and therefore injuries did not consistently increase in the presence of increasing acuity. Regardless of the reasons for this confounding finding, opportunities to further study SPHM in subacute settings exist, and should be taken as part of the strategic plan toward safer, more cost-efficient healthcare across practice settings.

Evidence for Standard 8: Some Resources and Readings

American Nurses Association. (2013). *Safe patient handling and mobility: Interprofessional national standards.* Silver Spring, MD: Nursesbooks.org.

American Physical Therapy Association (APTA). (2013, January 15). Early rehab in ICU generates net financial savings for hospitals. *PT in Motion: News Now.* Retrieved August 26, 2013, from http://www.apta.org/PTinMotion/NewsNow/2013/1/15/EarlyRehabStudy/

Cohen, M. A., Green, D. A., Nelson, G. G., Leib, R., Matz, M. A., et al. (2010). *Patient handling and movement assessments: A white paper* (Prepared by the 2010 Health Guidelines Revision Committee Specialty Subcommittee on Patient Movement). Dallas, TX: Facility Guidelines Institute. Retrieved August 7, 2013, from http://www.fgiguidelines.org/pdfs/FGI_PHAMA_whitepaper_042810.pdf

D'Arcy, L. P., Sasai, Y., & Stearns, S. C. (2012). Do assistive devices, training, and workload affect injury incidence? Prevention efforts by nursing homes and back injuries among nursing assistants. *Journal of Advanced Nursing, 68*(4), 836-845.

Edlich, R. F., Winters, K. L., Hudson, M. A., Britt, L. D., & Long, W. B. (2004). Prevention of disabling back injuries in nurses by the use of mechanical patient lift systems. *Journal of Long-Term Effectiveness of Medical Implants, 14*(6), 521-533.

ISHN Magazine. (2013). Health care industry must modernize patient lifting for safety's sake, says report. Retrieved June 22, 2013, from http://www.ishn.com/articles/96172-health-care-industry-must-modernize-patient-lifting-for-safetys-sake-says-report?WT.rss_f=Today%27s+News&WT.rss_a=Health+care+industry+must+modernize+patient+lifting+for+safety%E2%80%99s+sake%2C+says+report&WT.rss_ev=a

Marx, M. (2005). Six Sigma in the healthcare industry. Retrieved May 22, 2013, from http://www.isixsigma.com/industries/healthcare/six-sigma-healthcare-industry/

Mattei, S. Y. (2012, June). *A report to New Yorkers: The case for caring technology.* New York, NY: New Yorkers for Patient & Family Empowerment.

Park, R. M., Bushnell, P. T., Bailer, A. J., Collins, J. W., & Stayner, L. T. (2009). Impact of publicly sponsored interventions on musculoskeletal injury claims in nursing homes. *American Journal of Industrial Medicine, 52*(9), 683-697.

Pexton, C. (2010). *Healthcare quality initiatives: The role of leadership.* Retrieved May 22, 2013, from http://www.isixsigma.com/implementation/change-management-implementation/healthcare-quality-initiatives-role-leadership/

Pexton, C. (2005). *One piece of the safety puzzle: Advantages of the Six Sigma approach.* Retrieved May 22, 2013, from http://www.psqh.com/janfeb05/sixsigma.html

Pexton, C. (2005). *Overcoming barriers to change using Six Sigma.* Retrieved May 22, 2013, from http://www.isixsigma.com/implementation/change-management-implementation/overcoming-barriers-change-healthcare-system/

Policy and advocacy: Safe patient handling and mobility. (2010). Retrieved May 22, 2013, from http://nursingworld.org/MainMenuCategories/Policy-Advocacy/State/Legislative-Agenda-Reports/State-SafePatientHandling

Trinkoff, A. M., Muntaner, C., & Le, R. (2005). Staffing and worker injury in nursing homes. *American Journal of Public Health, 95*(7), 1220-1225.

Summary: A Vision for the Future

In summary, the term *safety culture* is a relatively recent idea, and appears to have arisen out of the 1986 Chernobyl disaster investigations and report, where violations of the operating procedures were thought to have contributed to the accident. A culture of safety is the way in which high-reliability industries such as aviation, nuclear power, oil and gas, and health care are moving forward to meet goals and objectives. The reason for this realignment with safety goals is that previously structured safety programs that relied on management to monitor safety simply do not work. A culture of safety relies on employee involvement, along with the practice of developing managers who support safety initiatives that include every member of the team.

SPHM is a driver of safety on many levels. Originally introduced as a method to manage worker's compensation costs, SPHM has become a strategy to manage risk across units, disciplines, and practice settings. As described in the SPHM Standards, features of a culture of safety include acknowledgment of the risk, a commitment to provide resources to consistently achieve safe operations, a blame-free environment where individuals are able to report errors or incidents without fear, and an emphasis on collaboration across sectors and settings.

Healthcare quality and safety have received intense scrutiny since the 1999 IOM report, *To Err Is Human: Building a Safer Health System* (Kohn, Corrigan, & Donaldson, 1999). Healthcare organizations have responded to this challenge, and many healthcare facilities are using NDNQI® to identify the structures and processes that improve safety and outcomes of care. A SPHM program may affect a variety of NDNQI measures. For instance, Sturman-Floyd reports that she found a relationship between ceiling lift systems and the reduction of pressure ulcer incidence. She noted that fewer staff members were needed to move healthcare recipients and that by using the technology, family members could turn and reposition the healthcare recipients at home between professional care visits.

Furthermore, as healthcare organizations respond to changes in reimbursement practices that focus on outcomes and cost, direct and indirect mobility-related outcomes become increasingly important. SPHM is addressing fiscal initiatives, which not only reduce injury of healthcare workers, but also improve safety of healthcare recipients. For example, consider Mercy Health in Missouri: Karin Garrett explains that length of stay among high-risk patients (patients of size) and fall-related injuries both have decreased there as awareness of the SPHM program increased (Garrett, 2013). Julie Lavezzo and Ryan Rodriguez (2013) experienced a similar data outcome with introduction of the mobility coach role to the SPHM program at Marin General Hospital (MGH). Further, at MGH, a qualitative study suggested profound satisfaction, expressed not only by healthcare workers, but by healthcare recipients as well. Darla Watanabe at Stanford Hospitals and Clinics explained that, like Sturman-Floyd, a reduction in the frequency and severity of hospital-acquired pressure ulcers has emerged alongside the maturing of the SPHM programs (Watanabe, 2013). The interprofessional nature of the SPHM Standards is emphasized throughout this document because the value of the Standards is dependent on recognizing how different units, disciplines, and settings interface. To achieve the highest level of success, it is important to understand the underlying causes behind immobility-related consequences of care—the adverse outcomes that are considered nonreimbursable events due to CMS payment restructuring. These underlying causes are often the failure of the healthcare worker to successfully lift, turn, and reposition dependent or immobile healthcare recipients. For the first time, healthcare workers, managers, and leaders have tools to address these underlying causes. The tools serve to assist the healthcare worker in providing early, progressive mobility while managing the risks of MSD and other injury. SPHM tools enhance the culture of safety by involving frontline healthcare workers and providing defined safety opportunities for manager and leader support over time. It is more important than ever to understand the value of a culture of safety as both healthcare recipients and workers are becoming older and larger, creating a "perfect storm" for costly catastrophic injuries in healthcare settings across the United States.

Although the prevalence of obesity in America fluctuates based on the location of data collection, study design, age of participants, and other factors, most researchers agree that nearly 40% of adult Americans living in the United States are obese, 67% are overweight or obese, and nearly 7% are considered morbidly obese. This increase in the prevalence of obesity is occurring at the same time the general population and healthcare worker population are both aging. For example, the proportion of Americans 65 years of age and older is expected to increase from 12% in 2005 to approximately 20% by 2030. In 2013, the age of the average nurse is 53. These parallel increases affect the ability of healthcare workers to manually lift, and concurrently the acuity of patients is also increasing. Sicker, more dependent healthcare recipients are presenting to larger, older healthcare workers. Again, meaningful SPHM strategies are at the heart of risk management associated with this emerging storm. To integrate the SPHM Standards into a meaningful culture of safety, the SPHM program must address safety issues irrespective of the etiology. A safe work environment and corresponding attitudes will succeed only if these qualities are pervasive across all units, disciplines, and practice settings.

Early, progressive mobility is an emerging trend in the United States and globally. The trend in healthcare today is early mobility. We recognize that this practice reduces not only hospital costs, but also post-acute costs. Cognitive function in the first year after hospitalization is also impaired after prolonged immobility. SPH is reflecting and supporting mobility practices and, even though we have used the term movement for the past decade or more, the focus of programs in the future will be safe patient handling and mobility. This growing interest is a result of quantifiable economic, clinical, and humanistic outcomes associated with early, progressive mobility. However, without strategies to promote safety in this practice, dangers surface among both healthcare workers and recipients. These dangers may be due to the nature of the healthcare recipients and workers, in that they may very well share the risks of being older and of size. SPHM prevents unanticipated immobility, and therefore the common, predictable, and preventable consequences of care.

Poor facility design may act as a barrier to implementing a SPHM program; yet resources are available that guide healthcare workers, managers, and leaders to effectively address such barriers. Education and training designed to address the needs of both healthcare recipients and workers can assist in creating a culture of safety that prevents error or disregard of safety because of accountability from both. Safety is the ability to fully integrate the patient-centered assessment and plan of care that incorporates use of SPHM technology and skills. Protecting injured healthcare workers further establishes the value the organization places on the long-term safety of the family of healthcare workers. Ongoing evaluation validates the overall efforts of a SPHM program. Consider each of the quality indicators as described herein that hold either a direct or an indirect relationship to SPHM. Successful healthcare workers, managers, and leaders seek to explore further outcome opportunities as programs mature and evolve. For example, qualitative findings that help to support the satisfaction efforts in an organization, and further link such scores to liability risk and disclosure opportunities, are examples of the indirect value of a SPHM program.

The opportunities associated with SPHM are endless. The key is to transform the SPHM program into a safety culture. The tools and resources are available. The challenge is to acknowledge health care as a high-reliability industry, recognize the need to realign SPHM with the overall safety goals of the organization, and seek frontline healthcare worker involvement that management and leadership economically and holistically support.

Evidence: Some Resources and Reading

Becher, E. C., & Chassin, M. R. (2001). Improving the quality of health care: Who will lead? *Health Affairs, 20*(5), 164-179.

Centers for Medicare and Medicaid Services (CMS). *Pressure ulcers.* Retrieved June 6, 2013, from http://partnershipforpatients.cms.gov/p4p_resources/tsp-pressureulcers/toolpressureulcers.html

Charney, W. (2011). *Handbook of modern hospital safety.* Boca Raton, FL: CRC Press.

Charney, W. (2012). *Epidemic of medical errors and hospital-acquired infections.* Boca Raton, FL: CRC Press.

Charney, W., & Schirmer, J. (2007). Nursing injury rates and negative patient outcomes—Connecting the dots. *AAOHN Journal, 5*(11), 1-6, 17.

Cohen, M. A., Green, D. A., Nelson, G. G., Leib, R., Matz, M. A., et al. (2010). *Patient handling and movement assessments: A white paper.* (Prepared by the 2010 Health Guidelines Revision Committee Specialty Subcommittee on Patient Movement.) Dallas, TX: Facility Guidelines Institute. Retrieved August 7, 2013, from http://www.fgiguidelines.org/pdfs/FGI_PHAMA_whitepaper_042810.pdf

Committee on Quality of Healthcare in America. (2001). *Crossing the quality chasm: A new health system for the 21st century.* Washington, DC: National Academies Press.

Flegal, K. M., Carroll, M. D., Ogden, C. L., & Curtin, L. R. (2010). Prevalence and trends in obesity among U.S. adults, 1999-2008. *Journal of the American Medical Association 303*(3), 235-241.

Frankel, A. S., Leonard, M. W., & Denham, C. R. (2006, August). Fair and just culture, team behavior, and leadership engagement: The tools to achieve high reliability. *Health Services Resource, 41*(4), 1690-1709.

Fryar, C., Carroll, M., & Ogden, C. (2012). *Prevalence of overweight, obesity, and extreme obesity among adults: United States, trends 1960-1962 through 2009-2010.* Retrieved June 6, 2013, from http://www.cdc.gov/nchs/data/hestat/obesity_adult_09_10/obesity_adult_09_10.pdf

Gallagher, S. M. (2011). Exploring the relationship between obesity, patient safety, and caregiver injury. *American Journal of SPHM, 1*(2), 8-12.

Gallagher, S. M., Steadman, A., & Gallagher, S. M. (2010). Tackling tough topics: Successful frontline conversations every time! *Bariatric Times, 7*(6), 1, 5-9.

Garrett, K. (2013). Personal communication/conversation with author, August 6, 2013.

Grenny, J. (2003). Crucial conversations: Where are you stuck? That's where a crucial conversation is waiting. Retrieved May 17, 2013, from http://findarticles.com/p/articles/mi_m0MNT/is_12_57/ai_n6108404/

Institute of Medicine. (2008). *Retooling for an aging America: Building the health care workforce.* Retrieved June 6, 2013, from http://www.iom.edu/Reports/2008/Retooling-for-an-Aging-America-Building-the-Health-Care-Workforce.aspx

Kohn, L., Corrigan, J., & Donaldson, M. (1999). *To err is human: Building a safer health system.* Washington, DC: National Academies Press.

Lavezzo, J., & Rodriguez, R. (2013). *Transforming a program into a culture: Exploring the role of the lift coach as the missing element to meaningful safe patient handling and mobility.* Rancho Mirage, CA: Southern California Association Health Risk Managers.

Leape, L. L., Berwick, D. M., & Bates, D. W. (2002). What practices will most improve safety? *Journal of the American Medical Association 288*(4), 501-507.

Mohr, J., & Batalden, P. B. (2002). Improving safety on the front lines: The role of clinical microsystems. *Quality & Safety in Healthcare, 11*, 45–50.

National Institute for Occupational Safety and Health. *NIOSH program portfolio: Musculoskeletal disorders.* Retrieved June 6, 2013, from http://www.cdc.gov/niosh/programs/msd/

National Patient Safety Foundation. (2013). *Through the eyes of the workforce: Creating joy, meaning, and safer health care.* Boston: Lucian Leape Institute at the NPSF.

National Quality Forum. *Effective communication and care.* Retrieved June 6, 2013, from http://www.qualityforum.org/Topics/Effective_Communication_and_Care_Coordination.aspx

Nelson, A., Collins, J., Siddarthan, K., Matz, M., & Waters, T. (2008). Link between safe patient handling and patient outcomes in long-term care. *Rehabilitation Nursing, 33*(1), 33-43.

Nelson, E. C., Batalden, P. B., & Huber, T. P. (2002). Microsystems in healthcare. Part 1. Learning from high-performing front-line clinical units. *Joint Commission Journal on Quality Improvement, 28*, 472–493.

Occupational Safety and Health Administration. *Healthcare facilities: Safe patient handling*. Retrieved June 6, 2013, from http://www.osha.gov/SLTC/healthcarefacilities/safepatienthandling.html

Patterson, K., Grenny, J., McMillan, R., & Switzler, A. (2005). *Crucial confrontations: Tools for resolving broken promises, violated expectations, and bad behavior*. New York: McGraw-Hill.

Pexton, C. (2005). *Healthcare quality initiatives: The role of leadership*. Retrieved May 22, 2013, from http://www.isixsigma.com/implementation/change-management-implementation/healthcare-quality-initiatives-role-leadership/

Pizzi, L., Goldfarb, N. I., & Nash, D. B. (2010). Crew resource management and its applications in medicine. In A. J. Markowitz (Ed.), *Making health care safer: A critical analysis of patient safety practices* (Agency for Healthcare Research and Quality Evidence Report/Technology Assessment No. 43). Retrieved from www.ahrq.gov/clinic/ptsafety/chap44.htm

Reducing nursing injuries. Retrieved June 1, 2013, from http://individual.utoronto.ca/anamjitsivia/nursesrfp.pdf

Rodriguez, R., & Lavezzo, J. (2013). *Uplifted: Giving voice to safe patient handling—Building a caregiver narrative*. Wilmington, DE: Association of Safe Patient Handling Professionals.

Schoenfisch, A. L., Pompeii, L. A., Myers, D. J., James, T., Yeung, Y., Fricklas, E., Pentico, M., & Lipscomb, H. J. (2011). Objective measures of adoption of patient lift and transfer devices to reduce nursing staff injuries in the hospital setting. *American Journal of Industrial Medicine, 54*(12), 935-945.

Singer, S. J., & Tucker, A. L. *Creating a culture of safety in hospitals*. Retrieved April 28, 2013, from http://iis-db.stanford.edu/evnts/4218/Creating_Safety_Culture-SSingerRIP.pdf

Sturman-Floyd, M. (2012). *Reducing the prevalence of pressure ulcers among bed bound patients*. Retrieved May 29, 2013, from www.slideshare.net/mha_nz/1400-1500-melanie-sturman-reducing-the-incidence-fri

Watanabe, D. (2013). Personal communication/conversation with author, August 10, 2013.

Appendix A. Sample SPHM Policies and Procedures

Safe Patient Handling and Mobility Sample Policy

PURPOSE

To establish a policy that ensures healthcare workers use safe patient handling and mobility principles to reduce the risk of injury to healthcare recipients and workers, and to maintain an environment of dignity, safety, trust, and comfort.

POLICY

Safe patient handling and mobility practices will be used in all areas of the organization, as described in this policy and corresponding procedures. The purpose of this policy is to ensure healthcare workers and recipients that safety is the organization's highest priority. To accomplish this, a safe patient handling and mobility (SPHM) program will be implemented and sustained in order to ensure required infrastructure is in place to comply with components of this program's underlying policy. The program will include a process for the worker's right to refuse to participate in activities unsafe for the healthcare worker or recipient. A nonpunitive policy will be in place to support a better understanding of risks and barriers to safety. This infrastructure includes an assessment process for healthcare recipients, facility assessment and design to support safe practices, assessment tools to identify and manage high-risk tasks, handling and mobility technology, program elements to support use of technology, creative meaningful worker training (unit-, discipline- or facility-specific training), relevant education, communication, and a commitment to transforming the program into a culture of safety.

DEFINITIONS

Assessment process for healthcare recipients. Use of a scoring or other system to examine and evaluate the physical, mental, cognitive, medical, and/or environmental conditions of a healthcare recipient to determine appropriate

SPHM methods, technology, and supplies. Assessment for SPHM may be an interprofessional activity, with collaboration from several disciplines.

Culture of safety. Core values and behaviors resulting from a collective and sustained commitment by organizational leadership, managers, and healthcare workers to emphasize safety over competing goals.

Healthcare worker. An individual involved in the provision of care to another individual and who works for the employer at any level in the continuum of care. Examples of healthcare workers include, but are not limited to, nurses, nursing assistants, resident assistants, home health aides, direct care workers working in community settings, occupational therapists, physical therapists, therapist assistants, radiology technologists, infection control practitioners, peer leaders, social workers, morgue personnel, emergency medical technicians, paramedics, and transporters, physicians, dentists, school teachers, and para-educators. Settings with organized labor should include union representation.

High-risk tasks. Patient handling and mobility tasks characterized by biomechanical and postural stressors imposed on the healthcare worker.

Mobility. Progressive and active maintenance of, or increase in, physical activity of a healthcare recipient with or without assistance of healthcare worker action and SPHM technology.

Nonpunitive environment. An environment that fosters trust to encourage healthcare workers to disclose healthcare errors so that the precursors to errors can be better understood and remedied. Healthcare workers know that they are accountable for their actions, but will not be held accountable for problems within the system or environment that are beyond their control.

Right of refusal. The right of the healthcare worker to refuse an assignment, or a healthcare recipient to refuse a treatment or the use of SPHM technology.

Safe patient handling and mobility (SPHM) program. A formal, systematized program for reducing the risk of injuries and MSDs for healthcare workers, fostering a culture of safety while improving the quality of care and reducing the risk of physical injury to healthcare recipients.

REFERENCES

American Nurses Association. *Safe patient handling and mobility: Interprofessional national standards.* Silver Spring, MD: Author.

Centers for Disease Control. *Safe Patient Handling: NIOSH Workplace Safety.* Accessed at: http://www.cdc.gov/niosh/topics/safepatient/

VISN 8 Patient Safety Center of Inquiry. *Facility Safe Patient Handling policy Draft: Draft of a safe patient handling and movement policy you can adapt for your facility.* Accessed at: http://www.visn8.va.gov/PatientSafetyCenter/safePtHandling/

The Joint Commission (TJC). (2012). *Improving patient and worker safety: Opportunities for synergy, collaboration and innovation.* Oakbrook Terrace, IL: The Joint Commission. Retrieved from http://www.jointcommission.org

University of Texas Medical Branch. *Guidelines for Safe Patient Handling and Movement.* Accessed at: www.utmb.edu/Policies_And_Procedures/Health_Safety_and_Security/...

Safe Patient Handling and Mobility Sample Procedure

PURPOSE

To identify and describe procedures that support a Safe Patient Handling and Mobility (SPHM) program, for purposes of promoting safe, dignified handling and mobility.

PROCEDURE

Safe patient handling and mobility procedures support the SPHM policy and describe actions which correspond with the policy.

Accountability and Responsibility of Healthcare Workers

I. Compliance
   a. It is the duty of healthcare workers to take reasonable care of their own health and safety, as well as that of their co-workers and health-care recipients during patient handling and mobility activities by following these procedures.
   b. Non-compliance with procedures will indicate a need for retraining and/or corrective action.

II. Patient Handling and Mobility Requirements
   a. All patients will be assessed to determine their handling and mobility needs, and how best to accomplish this in the safest way.
   b. Plan activities to avoid hazardous patient handling and mobility tasks whenever possible.
   c. Use technology such as mechanical lifting devices and other approved handling aids for handling and mobility tasks.
   d. Use technology such as mechanical lifting devices and other approved handling and mobility aids in accordance with instructions and training.

III. Education/Training
   a. Healthcare workers will complete and document education and training as required to ensure correct and proper use and understanding of safe patient handling and mobility principles and technology.

IV. Technology
   a. Mechanical lifting devices and other equipment/aids will be conveniently placed in locations for ease of access.
   b. Mechanical lifting devices and other equipment/aids will be maintained regularly and kept in proper working order.

V. Reporting of Musculoskeletal Disorders or other Injuries/Incidents
   a. Healthcare workers shall report to their supervisor all injuries from handling and mobility.

Accountability and Responsibility of Employers

I. Ensure high-risk tasks are assessed prior to activity and are completed safely, using appropriate technology

II. Ensure technology is available, maintained regularly, in proper working order, and stored conveniently and safely.

III. Ensure employees complete education and training as required for patient handling and mobility.

IV. Maintain training records as required by the facility.

V. Ensure workers have the right to refuse to perform or be involved in patient handling or mobility they believe in good faith will expose a healthcare worker or recipient to an unacceptable risk of injury.

VI. Refer all staff reporting injuries due to patient handling tasks.

VII. Maintain incident/injury reports and supplemental injury statistics as required.

Accountability and Responsibility of Interprofessional Team

I. Develop Interprofessional Team to support efforts for transforming a SPHM program into a SPHM Culture of Safety.

II. Education and Training department
   a. Assist with the annual training required to ensure workers stay competent with SPHM policies and procedures.
   b. Assure that all new employees are educated on the policy and procedures of moving, lifting, transferring and repositioning healthcare recipients.
   c. Coordinate on-going, on-unit or "Just-In-Time" Training

III. Engineering department
   a. Maintain mechanical SPHM technology in proper working order.
   b. Inspect and approve all incoming technology.
   c. Coordinate installation of technology.

IV. Ergonomics department
   a. Research and provide information regarding technology needed for the implementation of the SPHM program.

       b. Provide training to workers and others as needed.

   V. Infection Control

       a. Monitor processing of technology and devices

  VI. Laundry (Environmental Services)

       a. Process slings and other reusable devices

 VII. Nursing, Therapy, Ancillary/Support Staff, and Patient Care Services

       a. Establish a process for SPHM Assessment, which includes having healthcare recipients assessed for handling and mobility needs.

       b. Establish a process for Technology Needs Assessment to determine which handling aids/devices are most appropriate for each situation.

       c. Assess working environment and the potential barriers to utilizing technology by reducing the room clutter, or unsafe floor coverings.

       d. Encourage healthcare recipients to assist when possible with the move, lift, transfer or reposition.

       e. Document handling mobility needs on the plan of care.

       f. Document the technology used and the healthcare recipient's response to the move, lift, transfer or reposition.

       g. Participate directly or indirectly on the Safe Patient Handling Interprofessional Team, which could include but is not limited to; assisting with on-going hazard assessments, providing feedback to department representatives, and attending team meetings.

VIII. Facility design

       a. In planning new construction or remodeling of a patient care area, recognize the physical space and construction design needed to incorporate technology at a later date.

DEFINITIONS

Ancillary/support staff. Individuals whose work provides necessary support to the SPHM program. This may include consultants and staff members from departments such as risk management, safety, infection prevention, occupational health, transportation, security, activity direction, recreational therapy, creative art therapy, environmental services, laundry, volunteers, engineering, biomedical engineering, facilities, morgue, funeral home, purchasing, and contracting.

Assessment for SPHM. Use of a scoring or other system to examine and evaluate the physical, mental, cognitive, medical, and/or environmental conditions of a healthcare recipient to determine appropriate SPHM methods, technology, and supplies. Assessment for SPHM may be an interprofessional activity, with collaboration from several disciplines.

Culture of safety. Core values and behaviors resulting from a collective and sustained commitment by organizational leadership, managers, and healthcare workers to emphasize safety over competing goals.

Education. The transfer of information to others in order to raise awareness and increase understanding of the subject. Includes relaying of information during orientation and in-service education.

Employer. The healthcare organization, agency, system, corporation, business, or person(s) that employ or contract with the healthcare worker, at all levels of the continuum of care. The term organization is used interchangeably in these standards.

Healthcare worker. An individual involved in the provision of care to another individual and who works for the employer at any level in the continuum of care. Examples of healthcare workers include, but are not limited to, nurses, nursing assistants, resident assistants, home health aides, direct care workers working in community settings, occupational therapists, physical therapists, therapist assistants, radiology technologists, infection control practitioners, peer leaders, social workers, morgue personnel, emergency medical technicians, paramedics, and transporters, physicians, dentists, school teachers, and para-educators. Settings with organized labor should include union representation.

High-risk tasks. Patient handling and mobility tasks characterized by biomechanical and postural stressors imposed on the healthcare worker.

Interprofessional. Reliant on the overlapping knowledge, skills, and abilities of each professional team member. Interprofessionalism can drive synergistic effects by which outcomes are enhanced and become more comprehensive than a simple aggregation of the individual efforts of the team members.

Mobility. Progressive and active maintenance of, or increase in, physical activity of a healthcare recipient with or without assistance of healthcare worker action and SPHM technology.

Musculoskeletal disorder (MSD). An injury or disorder of the muscles, nerves, tendons, joints, or cartilage, and disorder of the nerves, tendons, muscles, and supporting structures of the upper and lower limbs, neck, and lower back that are caused, precipitated, or exacerbated by sudden exertion or prolonged exposure to physical factors such as repetition, force, vibration, or awkward posture. This definition specifically excludes conditions such as fractures, contusions, abrasions, and lacerations resulting from sudden physical contact of the body with external objects.

Nonpunitive environment. An environment that fosters trust to encourage healthcare workers to disclose healthcare errors so that the precursors to errors can be better understood and remedied. Healthcare workers know that they are accountable for their actions, but will not be held accountable for problems within the system or environment that are beyond their control.

Right of refusal. The right of the healthcare worker to refuse an assignment, or a healthcare recipient to refuse a treatment or the use of SPHM technology.

Safe patient handling and mobility (SPHM) program. A formal, systematized program for reducing the risk of injuries and MSDs for healthcare workers, fostering a culture of safety while improving the quality of care and reducing the risk of physical injury to healthcare recipients.

Technology. The assistive tools used, within the organization and at the point of care, to facilitate the healthcare worker's performance of SPHM tasks, thus minimizing the risk of injury to the healthcare recipient and the healthcare worker. Technology may include equipment, devices, accessories, software, and multimedia resources.

Technology needs assessment. An assessment done by using ergonomic principles of evaluation. The assessment includes evaluation of the physical, mental, and cognitive characteristics of the healthcare recipient or population, and the physical environment of care in which care is being delivered, so as to recommend appropriate SPHM methods and technology.

Training. The process of bringing a person to an agreed standard of proficiency by hands-on practice or simulation applications.

REFERENCES

American Nurses Association. *Safe patient handling and mobility: Interprofessional national standards.* Silver Spring, MD: Author.

Centers for Disease Control. *Safe Patient Handling: NIOSH Workplace Safety.* Accessed at: http://www.cdc.gov/niosh/topics/safepatient/

Charney, W. (2007). Nursing injury rates and negative patient outcomes: Connecting the dots. *AAOHN Journal, 55*(11), 470-475.

Gallagher SM. (2009). Patient transferring challenges. *Bariatric Times, 6*(4), 12-18.

The Joint Commission (TJC). (2012). *Improving patient and worker safety: Opportunities for synergy, collaboration and innovation.* Oakbrook Terrace, IL: The Joint Commission. Retrieved from http://www.jointcommission.org

Tullar, J. B. (2010). Occupational safety and health interventions to reduce musculoskeletal symptoms in the health care sector. *Journal of Occupational Rehabilitation 20*(2), 199-219.

University of Texas Medical Branch. *Guidelines for Safe Patient Handling and Movement.* Accessed at: www.utmb.edu/Policies_And_Procedures/Health_Safety_and_Security/...

VISN 8 Patient Safety Center of Inquiry. *Facility Safe Patient Handling policy draft: Draft of a safe patient handling and movement policy you can adapt for your facility.* Accessed at: http://www.visn8.va.gov/PatientSafetyCenter/safePtHandling/

VISN 8 Patient Safety Center of Inquiry. *Patient care slings selection and toolkit.* Retrieved from http://www.visn8.va.gov/visn8/Patientsafetycenter/safePtHandling/default.asp

VISN 8 Patient Safety Center of Inquiry. *Patient care ergonomics resource guide: Safe patient handling.* Retrieved from http://www.visn8.va.gov/patientsafetycenter/resguide/ErgoGuidePtOne.pdf

Waters, L. (2007). When is it safe to manually lift a patient? *American Journal of Nursing, 107*(8).

Right to Refuse Sample Policy and Procedure
PURPOSE
The purpose of the Right to Refuse policy and procedure is to protect the healthcare worker and recipient from unnecessary harm, alert the chain of command to the suspected harm, and trigger a quality investigation.

POLICY
No healthcare worker will be subject to disciplinary action for refusing to perform or be involved in handling or mobility tasks if the worker believes in good faith that the task will expose a healthcare worker or recipient to an unacceptable risk of injury as long as the worker, in good faith, follows the requirements set forth in this procedure.

PROCEDURE
In the event that a healthcare worker does refuse in good faith to participate in handling or mobility, he/she must do the following:

- Notify the supervisor or their designee (Chain of Command) immediately of the refusal and the reason for doing so.
- Stay on the job and make him/herself available to the supervisor in the event the suspected unsafe situation can be resolved.
- If called to assist with a healthcare recipient who is in distress, the worker will remain with the healthcare recipient as necessary, providing assistance as able until the necessary resources are available.
- Complete the appropriate After Action Review process.

DEFINITIONS
Healthcare worker. An individual involved in the provision of care to another individual and who works for the employer at any level in the continuum of care. Examples of healthcare workers include, but are not limited to, nurses, nursing assistants, resident assistants, home health aides, direct care workers working in community settings, occupational therapists, physical therapists, therapist assistants, radiology technologists, infection control practitioners, peer leaders, social workers, morgue personnel, emergency medical technicians, paramedics, and transporters, physicians, dentists, school teachers, and para-educators. Settings with organized labor should include union representation.

Healthcare recipient. An individual who is receiving health care. In the context of these standards, they are individuals who are receiving health care that involves assistance with handling and mobility. This definition is inclusive of patients, clients, residents, students, individuals living in community settings, and others as appropriate. Patient families and volunteer caregivers are included.

After action review. An after-action review (AAR) is a professional discussion of an event, focused on performance standards, that enables individuals or Committee members to discover for themselves what happened, why it happened, and how to sustain strengths and improve on weaknesses. It is a tool leaders and units can use to get maximum benefit from every task.

REFERENCES

American Nurses Association. *Safe patient handling and mobility: Interprofessional national standards.* Silver Spring, MD: Author.

Centers for Disease Control. *Safe Patient Handling: NIOSH Workplace Safety.* Accessed at: http://www.cdc.gov/niosh/topics/safepatient/

Cooper, M, D. (2000). Toward a model of safety culture. *Safety Science 36*: 111-136

The Joint Commission (TJC). (2012). *Improving patient and worker safety: Opportunities for synergy, collaboration and innovation.* Oakbrook Terrace, IL: The Joint Commission. Retrieved from http://www.jointcommission.org

United States Air Force. *The After Action Review.* Accessed at: http://www.au.af.mil/au/awc/awcgate/army/tc_25-20/chap1.htm

University of Texas Medical Branch. *Guidelines for Safe Patient Handling and Movement.* Accessed at: www.utmb.edu/Policies_And_Procedures/Health_Safety_and_Security/...

VISN 8 Patient Safety Center of Inquiry. *Facility Safe Patient Handling Policy draft: Draft of a safe patient handling and movement policy you can adapt for your facility.* Accessed at: http://www.visn8.va.gov/PatientSafetyCenter/safePtHandling/

Index

A

Alternative work in return to work, 76

American Nurses Association, 1, 4, 5

National Database of Nursing Quality Indicators (NDNQI), 5, 32, 70, 84, 85, 91

Agency for Healthcare Research and Quality (AHRQ), 5

Assessment, care planning, and technology use (Standard 6), 30–32, 65–73

assessment tools, 48, 66, 67, 68, 69

assisted living facility setting, 72–73

baseline assessment, 29, 48

communication in, 65, 67, 68, 69, 70, 71

data collection, 67, 68, 70, 71

delegation, 67, 71, 72

documentation in care plan, 68

healthcare recipients in, 65–66, 67, 68, 70, 71

mobility assessment, 48, 66, 67, 68, 69

patient-centered care and, 65

organizational assessment, 49

of SPHM programs, 27

SPHM technology and, 48, 67, 68

Standard 6 implementation, 67–73

transitions of care, 68–69, 72

See also Employer implementation; Healthcare worker implementation (Standard 6)

C

Care plans and planning and SPHM, 65

data collection, 68

documentation, 68

mobility assessment and, 68

SPHM technology and, 65, 68

transitions of care, 68–69, 72

See also Assessment, care planning, and technology use

Certification in SPHM, 5

Collaboration. *See* Communication and collaboration

Communication and collaboration

assessment and care planning and, 65, 67, 68, 69, 70, 71

care plans and, 68

communication of data, 67, 68, 70, 71

culture of safety and, 19–20, 22–23

with healthcare recipient, 71

reports and reporting, 17, 2, 31, 50, 53–54, 78, 84, 85

SPHM technology and, 47–48

Community settings considerations

assisted living facility (Standard 6), 72–73

employer-vendor resources (Standard 5), 63

home care (Standard 1), 23

home care (Standard 4), 54–55

long-term care research (Standard 8), 88

long-term care, rural (Standard 7), 79

rehabilitation center (Standard 3), 45

school-aged children, (Standard 2), 23

Competence and competencies in SPHM, 18, 33, 37, 61

See also Education, training, and maintaining competence

Culture of sacrifice, 1, 2, 91, 94

Culture of safety, 13–14

culture of safety and 19–20

employer commitment, 15–16

healthcare worker commitment, 20–22

home care setting, 23

setting up, 26–27

Standard 1 implementation, 14–23

See also Employer implementation; Healthcare worker implementation (Standard 1)